The Face of the Deep
Healing Body and Soul

Penny Allen

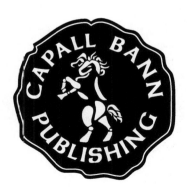

The Face of the Deep
Healing Body and Soul

©1998 Penny Allen

ISBN 186163 0409

Internal illustrations by the author, based on originals
Cover design by Paul Mason

Published by:

Capall Bann Publishing
Freshfields
Chieveley
Berks
RG20 8TF

Contents

Introduction   1

Nought   The Void   The Thalamus   5

One   The Sun   The Pineal   15

Two   The Moon   The Pituitary   24

Three   Mercury   The Thyroid   38

Four   Venus and the Earth   The Heart   50

Five   The Sun   The Solar Plexus   64

Six   Mars   The Hara   76

Seven   Jupiter   The Crown   85

Eight   Saturn   The Root   102

Nine   Uranus   The Mental Aura   114

Ten   Pluto   The Medulla   128

Eleven   Neptune   The Aura   143

Twelve   The Moon's Nodes   Enlightenment   163

Glossary   174

Further Reading   179

Introduction

Throughout recorded history there have been two traditions of thought: the orthodox and the heretical. Perhaps our current age is one of those historical moments when the division can break down and mainstream and alternative views can be seen for the unity they really are.

Scratch the surface of the New Age and you find beliefs that could be called conservative; delve into the orthodox and you find theories and practices that seem to be based more on superstition than on reason. Alternative remedies are usually the most ancient and traditional medical practice changes by the minute as new equipment and medicines are introduced.

There is no more a genuine division between the traditional and the alternative than there is between scientific and spiritual understanding, and to try to promote intuition over logic or vice versa is to create imbalance in our worlds and in ourselves. Just as we have two hemispheres of our brains, so we have access both to intuition and logic; we each have our share of reason and imagination and our share of faith and doubt. Without faith we would not get up in the mornings; without doubt we would not ask questions.

The healer who believes one hundred per cent in the process of healing is a rare and wondrous being. Most people who have experienced either the giving or receiving of healing spend most of their time doubting it and many of us, even those who should know better, spend quantities of energy and time in resisting it.

Every time I draw an astrological chart I think, 'What nonsense, how can this possibly work?' and every time I give the subsequent reading I am amazed and awe-struck by the fact that it does work. And when, despite my own reluctance, I find myself practising healing, I am always surprised: sometimes by the sheer force of the energy which may feel like a very fast current of air or intense cold or light, sometimes by the gentleness of imagery and colour that may appear either as inner vision or as a flash of vibrancy in the outer world, and I am always impressed by the courage and beauty of the human spirit as the individual's life journey unfolds. Similarly, in watching people in meditation, the first thing I have to do is acknowledge my own doubt - I know for sure that I am not going to attune to anything that is going to happen and am convinced that nothing is going to happen. Only then, with no expectations at all, is there a possiblity that I will get a glimpse of a person's story and of the help and guidance they may need.

Like many other people, I spend enormous amounts of energy and time refusing to do the thing that makes me well and happy and that also may have the benefit of helping other people.

What are we all afraid of? Ridicule, rejection, misunderstanding, hostility, and, more than that, we are afraid of what we might actually be doing, what powers we might be tapping into and encouraging. We are afraid, in short, of the Unknown.

These are genuine fears. Since classical times, people who have worked with the mysteries have been treated with suspicion with the effect that they have become isolated and the mysteries have become yet more mysterious. To understand the mysteries requires balance. They demand that you honour both your faith and your doubt, both your intuitive and your logical abilities. You cannot learn about healing, astrology or any alternative subject without practising it. To study astrology is to be an astrologer and to practise healing is to be a healer. That is all the qualification necessary. There is no distinction between the professional and the amateur, the public and the private.

For years I worked with astrology and healing knowing there were connections between them but not understanding what they were. In taking on the task of writing a book, I hoped that I would grasp what I could until then only intuitively sense. I could see there were links between the planets that continually move through our solar system and the chakras, or inner wheels, that continuously rotate in our bodies. Both are known as gods and even in our secular age newly discovered planets and other heavenly bodies are still named after deities and other mythological figures.

In the process of writing in what at first seemed a logical, causal way, I became aware of other themes: the attempt to link chakras and the endocrine glands with which they are associated to the planets drew in their related numbers and colours and, as I went from one chapter to the next I saw that the development of the human being bore a resemblance to that of the solar system itself and to other forms of life, in particular to the metamorphosis of the flying insect and its partner, the flower.

As I thought and wrote, I saw that the initial division from unity, described in so many myths as the separation or the fall, meant that everything was a reflection of everything else, a chip, as it were, off the same old block and I was reminded of the hermetic adage, As above, so below which seemed also to mean As within, so without, As over here, so over there, and As with me, so with you.

It became obvious that these correspondences were well known in ancient times when the mysteries had not been relegated to the heretical and alternative but were the focus for all the activities and thinking of society. This book is an attempt to get back to the roots of our own society as well as to the foundations of our bodies and personalities, and thereby to see our current beliefs and behaviour in the context of the past, a process which, I hope, may help point the way to a richer and more harmonious future.

I summon to the winding ancient stair,
Set all your mind upon the steep ascent,
Upon the broken, crumbling battlement,
Upon the breathless starlit air,
Upon the star that marks the hidden pole;
Fix every wandering thought upon
That quarter where all thought is done:
Who can distinguish darkness from the soul?

W B Yeats

Nought

The Void   The Thalamus

'Trace a circle no larger than a dot, the birth of eternal nature is therein contained'

Jakob Bohme

It was my first day at art school.

"Take a sheet of paper", said the teacher, "and break up the space" and he disappeared into a stock room.

No-one spoke. We didn't even look at each other. Everyone fixed their rectangles of paper to their easels, dipped brushes in paint and set to. But I was not going to be fooled by such a simple trick. I stood back and watched the other students. I am sure they were not really wearing berets and brandishing palettes but their confident flourishes suggested they should be. I, however, was not going to compete. I dipped my brush in black paint and made a tiny line in the centre of the page. Then I sat back and waited.

The students stole glances at each other while continuing to fill their paper with every conceivable colour and shape. I folded my arms and contemplated what the teacher might be doing in the stock room. Time ticked by. The students were adding splashes and squares, flecks and stars to their packed compositions.

I panicked. Memories came back of teachers scolding me for 'dreaming' as if doing nothing were the height of sin. Here I was wasting time while all these bright young things were producing real pictures. I took red paint and covered the page with it. I added some blue and some yellow and, by the time the teacher re-appeared, I had made an adequate semblance of a 'picture'. The teacher ambled round the room, his air of disdain withering our youthful pride. Then he sighed and said, "But all you had to do was one dot".

•

We had given him licence to punish us and, for the rest of that term, he did. In his lessons we were only allowed to make pictures with little circles of wood dipped in black paint. It was infuriating! We were young, creative, enthusiastic, longing to produce works of art that would stun the world and bring us our fortunes.

But I now appreciate his purpose; he was trying to show us the need for concentration and discipline and the importance of returning to the source of all forms. We had to learn to let go of competitiveness and to reach into some universal centre beyond the individual ego. I came to understand that, if I had simply made one dot on the paper and sat back in silence and confidence, I could have found not only my own centre but my own perimeter. Every dot or point has its aura or atmosphere just as a stone dropped in water produces circles. In being centred, one can move beyond the self-consciousness and concern about what others think to a genuine awareness of them. The circle is not destroyed by comparison and competition. If you focus on the dot at the centre, the circle will expand to contain everything and everyone.

A circle round a central point is a wheel. In Sanskrit (the Latin of the East) the word for wheel is *chakra*. In India, the word chakra is used a lot. There is nothing mysterious or esoteric about it: if you are feeling hot and bothered, you say, 'I'm in a real chakra today!'. Our equivalent is 'flat spin'. Wheels spin, their spokes rattle, the wind whistles through them. They go from A to B and back without knowing why and with no sense of progress. In the East, life is thought of as a wheel. We go round and round in a state of confusion, getting nowhere.

But in every wheel there is a little black dot, the still point at the centre and it is through that dot that one reaches calm and the possibility of viewing the confusion of the wheel from a state of detachment. Chakras, or wheels, are found in everything and, through their rotations, provide the energy for life.

My art teacher must have been drawing on great reserves of self-control to stop himself coming back into the Art Room. His purpose was to let us learn from our own purposelessness. He wanted us to discover for ourselves the importance of focus and concentration through the symbol of the single black dot.

The little black dot, which appears to be nothing, is, in fact, everything. It is the black hole that swallows suns, galaxies, universes. It is the tunnel of death, the birth canal and the fathomless well. The little black dot gives rise to consciousness itself; it is the pupil of the eye which absorbs information from the outer world and transforms it, by means of its negative, into imagery. My art teacher was trying to teach his pupils the meaning of the pupil.

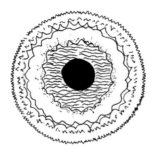

One of a stages used in the creation of the Universe (from an illustration of Robert Fludd's. 1617)

The word 'pupil' used to refer not to middle class children privileged enough to continue their education on state grants as we were then in the sixties. A pupil was an orphan, a child who was given an education with its keep. A pupil could make no choices; akin to pupil are words like 'puppet', 'puppy' and the French, 'poupée', or doll. The purpose of the pupil was to absorb information. Only later would the pupil be free to make decisions and display its imagination.

'Pupil' comes from the Latin *pupus* meaning 'boy'. The feminine, *pupa*, means both girl and an insect in chrysalis form. Girl and chrysalis are undergoing a process of transformation from which they will emerge as nymphs. A 'nymph' is both a beautiful young woman and a fully-formed winged insect. Desirable but unobtainable, nymphs are always on the move,

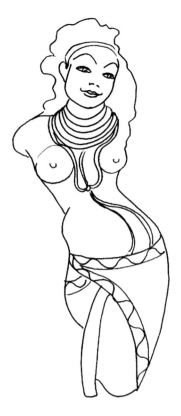

Tree nympth, India 9th century

slipping away from their pursuers. They cause nympholepsy in men who
lust after them and nymphomania in nymphs possessed by their own power.

Nymphs have been celebrated throughout the ages. One of the most famous
nymphs in history is Persephone or Kore whose name means 'maiden',
'bride' and 'the pupil of the eye'. The most famous nymph of twentieth
century fiction must surely be Lolita, who, having only just emerged from
her pupa or puberty, is trapped and, we would now say, 'sexually abused'
by her stepfather. Her creator, Vladimir Nabokov, was not only one of the
greatest novelists of the twentieth century but one of the greatest

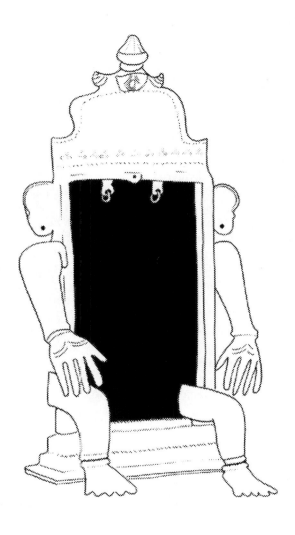

A bronze statue of the Goddess as the Void with space to hang her image.
India 19th century.

lepidopterists. A lepidopterist is a person who catches butterflies; his torture of the fully-formed insect, literally pinning it down into its death, masquerades as science but his main object is to fix the ephemeral in time, to prevent the nymph going through her next process of transformation. Lolita's stepfather is only attracted to young girls and finds his middle-aged wife disgusting in her womanhood. But, like everything else, Lolita must grow old and, by the end of the story, she is pregnant, poor and exhausted. Lolita's stepfather projects his own self-loathing, his fear of death and decay, onto the world around him, destroying the very people he has loved in his attempt to stay the movement of time.

The process of transformation involves darkness: one thing dies for another to be born. Darkness, black, absorbs and contracts. It provides the comfort of seclusion while one is going through change, whether mourning the loss of someone else or of a part of oneself. Black takes the light and vibrancy from any colour (as I told my teenage daughter when she begged me to let her paint her room black). And it takes a hell of a lot of white to lighten black (as I found out after my daughter had left home). Black turns matter into anti-matter, it swallows and devours, sucking everything towards it. It is hypnotic and magnetic, it is night and death; in black there is no identity.

Though black may be very small, it is highly concentrated. It is the common denominator in which everything returns to nothing. Black is dominant: the genes that produce dark hair, eyes and skin take precedence over those responsible for fairer colouring. White indeed is that which can withstand black dye, said Confucius. Add black to any colour and you get black.

Like black, nought is also dominant. Multiply any number by nought and the result will be nought. Within black are all the colours, undetectable because their light has gone; and within nought are all the numbers in their negative forms. Nought is the void, the end of everything and the beginning. It is not only death and the loss of identity but the pool, the source of all life. The void, the well, the pool, the source are all watery.

'In the beginning God created the heaven and the earth', Genesis tells us. 'And the earth was without form, and void; and darkness was upon the face of the deep: and the Spirit of God moved upon the face of the waters.' Black waters are a mirror, reflecting positive into negative through the shiny silver of their still surface. The silver of mirrors is made by painting black onto the back of a sheet of glass. A mirror, like the pupil of the eye or a camera, changes one thing into its image through reversal or negation.

The mirror is a doorway into another world. Behind it is anti-matter, shadow and negative forms, a world we can only access when we leave our conscious selves behind. Orpheus passed through it into the Underworld and Alice went through both the looking glass and the black tunnel of the rabbit's burrow into a world where meaning was topsy-turvy. Some of us seem to have easier access to it than others. My daughter, another Alice, is left-handed and, though she learned to write very easily, her writing could only be read if you held it to a mirror. Not only was every letter back to front but every line as well. Alice assures me she is in good company: Leonardo, Picasso and Goya, she says, did the same.

Mirrors and cameras never lie: they tell you who is the fairest of them all but, even if the answer is 'you', it will only be so for a time. Mirrors, like death, are great levellers - they reduce everything to nothing. And it is only through nothing that one can emerge again transformed. When we look into the mirror, the pool, the void or the source, we see ourselves. When God created the world from 'the waters of the deep', he looked at it after every stage and 'saw that it was good'. In other words, he was reflected back to himself in the void and saw that he was God. The face of the deep when made conscious is the face of God.

A circle, or nought, has no beginning or end and the black hole is both the tunnel of death which submerges personality and identity, and the source, the womb, the Great Mother from which all identities emerge. We come from the female, the black and the negative, and all of us, in our beginnings, are female. Both males and females carry the X chromosome and the Y chromosome only develops in the male foetus at a later stage. Behind the fear of women, black people, Jews (the original or 'Semite' race), gypsies, wolves, forests, dark and night is a terror of death, of losing identity in the great pool of negativity. Misogyny, racism and the systematic torture of animals in the name of science and nutrition develop from a fear of the mysterious unknown, and are a desperate attempt to cling to the rock of identity in the great waters of the void.

Thought itself can be seen as the emergence of air and light from the pool of the unconscious. So, not surprisingly, great philosophies and religions extol the male, the white and the dry as pure and supreme and the schools and churches in which they have been taught and practised have excluded people on the grounds of their colour, race and sex. The temples and churches from which women have been excluded exist outside the home and must often be reached by pilgrimage. The male worships through going out into the world of other males. The practice of worship for him, like trade and politics, takes place beyond the home.

In recent times women have hammered at the doors of the temples and institutes of education and the bastions of economic and political power and, in some places, some doors have opened a chink. But most doors remain firmly closed. Men sense that to open the doors to women is to open their systems and practices of belief to change. They are right. The first thing that women priests did on their inauguration in one English diocese was to join hands and dance in the cathedral.

Women's life experience is not the same as men's. Beliefs and spiritual practices develop around life experience. If it is possible to integrate the female understanding of the universe into traditional male practice, that practice will inevitably be altered. In the past, it was clearly understood that the ways of women and of men were different and necessitated different practices. Men developed their centres of worship, study, trade and politics outside the home, while women developed their culture inside.

Perhaps every culture in the world built itself originally around a central women's room, a symbolic womb. Such centres still exist in many places. In some societies they are beautifully decorated round huts and in others the womens quarters are the inner recesses of the house. It is out of the question for men to enter. It is a place where women go during menstruation and childbirth, it is where new life is brought into the world and nurtured and it is a place of ritual, worship and thanksgiving. It is known in English by the Greek word, *thalamus* or the Latin *gynaecium*.

The thalamus has traditionally been respected and protected as the heart of the culture's life, the centre of gestation, birth and nourishment as well as of wisdom, healing and magical practice. It constantly informs and guides the life that continues outside it. Outer and inner have been seen as symbolic states, the outer identified with consciousness, reason and worldly influence, while the inner requires a movement beyond consciousness, to areas of creative gestation, dream and the development of the psychic and intuitive powers.

It is easier to see what the male practice has been. Not only are male institutions publicly dominant, they have also relied on the written word, on the patronage of the arts, and on public ceremonies. Women's practice, however, has taken place in secret areas into which men, and, by extension, the conscious mind and the written word, were, by force of long tradition, not permitted entrance. Women's recent struggle to find acceptance in the male tradition has been necessitated by the destruction and domination of their hallowed practices and sacred temples.

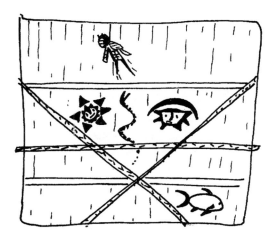

A wall of a hut in which girls retreat during the initiation rituals of puberty. Amazon. 20th century.

A meditation exercise

To start the process of meditation it is necessary to develop the means to sit still and concentrate. This is the most difficult part of the practice. To discipline oneself to sit alone and protected from disturbance for ten minutes each day is the best way to start.

> Place an object in front of you: a shell, stone, flower or candle or anything you have a feeling for.

Sit comfortably with your back as straight as possible and look at the object.

Thoughts will inevitably continue to pester your mind, attempting to distract you. But do not fight them. Keep bringing your attention back to the object and, in time, the thoughts will merge into the meditation.

One

The Sun   The Pineal

'If you throw a stone into the water, it becomes the centre and cause of many circles'

Leonardo da Vinci

The pupil of the eye is a deep dark well, a hole or tunnel that transforms one thing into its opposite. All animals are aware of its magnetic and hypnotic power but none more, perhaps, than reptiles. I discovered this one Easter Saturday when, walking on a cliff in Devon under a bright new Sun, I came upon a snake skin lying across my path. As I bent down, wondering whether to pick it up, I came eye to eye with the owner of the skin coiled beside it. It must have been an adder, its zigzags a sharp black and white due to the recent shedding of the skin.

It had fixed me with its stare and I straightened up unable to take my gaze from its shining black eye. We went on looking at each other like lovers or combatants until, eventually, I glanced up at the Sun which seemed to be a third party to our tryst and when I looked back the snake had gone.

Staring eyes have the power to benumb, the power of the narcotic. The narcissus flower is so called because of its numbing effects that cause a drowsiness as if induced by drugs. And the self-loving Narcissus was transfixed by his own reflection, like a drug addict deep into his own private fantasy. The drug-taker's hold on reality is shaky because he is unable to take his eyes off himself. His self-absorption pulls him into the vortex of his own soul and he drowns in his own negativity.

Narcissus was fixated on his own eye or I; his vanity made him conscious only of himself. Many nymphs fell in love with him but he would not give

15

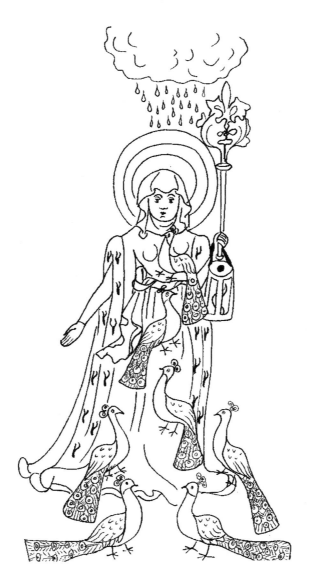

The Goddess, Iris surrounded by halo of the rainbow and peacocks.
Europe. 15th centruy.

them the time of day, obsessed as he was with his own loveliness. He simply sat and watched his own blue eye reflected in the crystal pool. (We know his eye was blue because, according to Robert Graves in *Greek Myths*, the narcissus is also the blue iris). What Narcissus saw in the pool was an iris surrounding a pupil, a circle round a central dot, the ancient symbol for the Sun, the golden egg or ego. Narcissus could go no further than number one; he was paralysed with an addiction for himself.

Not so God. When he looked into the pool of his own eye and 'saw that it was good', he didn't get trapped in the negativity of self love but took positive action. 'Let there be light', he commanded. The universe had started icy. Like all the best parties it took time to warm up. Before there was any light or sound the waters of the deep must have been extremely cold and dark. 'The face of the deep is frozen', God tells Job when describing his creation of the world.

God commanded the light into being through the medium of sound. The tumultuous tempest that arose from the thunder of his almighty voice and the lightning that he summonsed caused the ice to shatter into crystals. The effect of light shining on shattered ice is to divide it into prismatic colour. Where there is light there is also heat. Heat melts ice and causes vapour to rise. We tend to think, in our logical, causal way, that the Big Bang happened just once, somewhere out there in the universe and that it has little to do with us now. But perhaps the Big Bang is an ongoing process. Perhaps the void is with us always and is continually being shattered. Perhaps it is not only out there somewhere in the universe but in our minds and bodies. The Dalai Lama may have had a point when, to the question, 'What do you think about the Big Bang?', he answered, 'Which one?'.

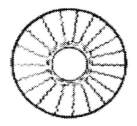

The effect of God's spirit moving on the face of the void was to bring into being the crystal, or iris. The iris is not only a beautiful blue flower but the wheel of the eye, the rainbow and, according to the Oxford English Dictionary 'a hexagonal prismatic crystal' while behind the iris of the eye lies the 'crystalline lens'. Crystal is said in esoteric teachings to be formed by the action of sound and light.

You could even say that crystal was the son of God: Christ or Krishna. It is used in computers and sound systems because it has the ability to hold masses of information. Not surprisingly, it has a memory that goes back to the beginnings of the universe. Crystal appears to be conscious and gives the impression of knowing everything. I once had a doll with blue glass eyes that looked like diamonds. When I wanted to do anything I thought she might disapprove of I had to turn her face to the wall. My doll was called Louise but she should have been called Iris.

Iris, the crystal, is the goddess of the rainbow, carrying information from the Source to the world of humanity, through the medium of colour. Among the innumerable odd inventions of the Victorians was a device called the iriscope. This was a piece of highly polished black glass which, when breathed on, released primary colours. The effect of breath on cold glass is to cause vapour and it is through vapour, or water, that colour shows. The Greeks have many words meaning breath or wind: one is *haliosis*, one is *zephyr*, and another is *aura*.

The aura is the atmosphere that surrounds and contains an entity. Humans have them, as do plants, as does the Earth itself. Like the atmosphere of the Earth, the human aura often goes unnoticed and, perhaps because of this, both are easily polluted. The aura is a breath or a breeze, a bubble of air containing water, the medium through which colour shows. It is the pull of the curve of the Earth's atmosphere that causes light to divide into colour and show the rainbow and the same is true of the human aura. Colours show through the action of light on water but they usually go unseen, lost in the blue-grey of the Earth's atmosphere but when the atmosphere of Earth is taken away, it is easy to see the aura around the human being.

There is no atmosphere on the Moon so the astronauts who landed there carried bottled oxygen and wore suits and golden helmets to protect them from the Sun's rays. I do not think the mission had in mind the desire to prove the existence of the human aura but an interesting aspect of the lunar landings was the rather comical blue atmosphere that surrounds the astronauts in the photographs.

Comedy was not, however, part of the show. The first Moon landing, on July 21st 1969, was as serious as the World Cup and the audience watching the television in the students' union to which I belonged was indistinguishable from a rugby crowd. I had gone from Art School to university but, like so many women, I found my education was predominantly in matters emotional rather than intellectual and at the time of the Moon landing I had just taken advantage of the new Abortion Act. (An extraordinary number of 'liberal' bills coincided with man's first steps on the Moon: bills regarding, for instance, divorce and homosexuality.)

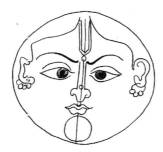

Solar mandala. India. 19th century.

It was impossible to find a seat in the packed room. I stood at the back and watched the crowd. There were very few women and the men were drinking beer, making fist salutes and shouting with excitement. I slunk away, vague questions forming in my mind: why was the rocket that went to the Moon called Apollo, god of the Sun? Why was the mission presented as a spectator sport? Why did the spacemen stick a flagpole in the surface of the Moon? Why did the flag represent a nation rather than the whole of humanity? Who was going to see and recognise the flag? And why had I had an abortion?

The Sun is an eye. An 'eye' is not only what we see with but is the central pivot of a system. And an eye represents consciousness itself. Light from the Sun beats like a pulse and the eye responds to it with a motion of contraction and dilation. The Sun is symbolised by a dot within a circle.

It shows consciousness, the simultaneous motion of contraction and expansion, which according to my daughter, Polly, is the fundamental motion of the universe. When Polly was three years old she used to beg me to stay by her bed at night in order to discuss the cosmos.

'What would happen if an ant lived on a volcano and the volcano erupted?' was one question that bothered her over many nights. 'Could the ant escape? Can an ant run faster than lava?' She did not want reassurance or pat answers. It would not do to say, 'The ant would be fine. It would run home to its Mummy and Daddy and have a nice mug of cocoa and go to bed.' What she wanted was the truth. Like so many children, she lay awake wondering how the universe began and what it was for. And sometimes she came to some interesting conclusions.

One night she said, 'Mum, you know there are only two things in the universe.' 'Yes?' I said. 'What are they?' 'In and out', she answered. I think she might have been right. In and out are the pump, the pulse, the breath, the heart beat, the contraction and dilation of birth, as well as of the pupil of the eye. The dot within the circle shows the movement of in/out, it is the symbol of potential and suggests many forms of life: the germ in the yolk, the nucleus in the atom, the tadpole in the spawn, the cycle of the Earth around the Sun and the Sun around the Earth.

The Sun's cycle provides the basis of time: the original clock is the sundial which measures the movement of the Sun around the Earth in twenty-four hours. In French, the word for time, *le temps*, also means weather. It relates to beat as in 'tempo' and to mood and atmosphere as in 'tempest', 'temperament' and 'temperature'. The incarnating soul, the pupil of the eye, is surrounded by the circle of its life and times, its destiny, its atmosphere or aura.

The pupil has been known as the 'mirror of the soul' and the pineal gland in the centre of the head was called by the philosopher Descartes 'the seat of the soul'. The pineal is our inner timepiece, our sundial or clock. It is responsible for the intake of light and is deeply sensitive to variations of light and dark. It gives us our sense of night and day and orients us not only in time but in space, providing the awareness of the four directions in relation to magnetic north. In fish the pineal is a huge gland giving direction in the depths of the ocean. In humans it releases the hormone melanin that causes tanning and protects from the rays of the Sun.

Providing orientation in time and space, it also gives us our awareness of the seasons and greater cycles of time. Through it, we attune to shifts in the weather. The pineal is so called because of its shape which is like a pine cone. The pine cone, too, dilates and contracts in relation to the weather. A diagram of the Sun, the circle with its central dot, when extended and shown from the side, looks like a trumpet of sound, a beam of light, or a cone. This is also how a chakra can be depicted sideways on.

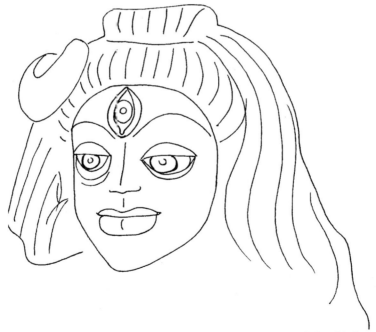

The Hindu god, Shiva, with the crescent Moon in his hair and the third eye on his forehead.

The pineal chakra is situated within the head but it can be contacted on the forehead and is often represented as the third or single eye. The single eye opens when the functions of the two physical eyes come into balance. The two eyes relate to the two glands in the centre of the head: the right to the pineal and the left to the pituitary, which in turn have a relationship to the Sun and the Moon, to gold and silver.

The ring around a central dot shows the rotation of the Earth around the Sun, a cycle of time. Add more rings and you get more cycles, an image that looks like the cross-section of a tree trunk (a pine perhaps).

The rotation of the Earth around the Sun takes place in one year and each ring of a tree trunk marks one year of its life. The rings of the tree are used not only to measure the age of the tree but to understand the temperature and weather conditions at any time in its history.

Rings are produced by dropping a stone in water. They ripple out to the edge and back again as an undertow. A ring could be described as the first movement, created by a stirring of the void, a movement that can be seen as a breath or aura, as a corona or halo of light, and as a vibration of sound which also is registered as a ring: we 'ring' bells which tell or toll the time. A bell and a clock were once one and the same and *la cloche* in French, confusingly, does not mean clock but bell.

Sun and Moon create the balance of night and day, heat and moisture, summer and winter. Without that balance there would be no growth, no life, no death. An over-concentration of Sun or consciousness, the urge for information at any cost, upsets the balance and causes damage to the element of water, the element associated with the subconscious. Apollo has no place on the Moon. Too much consciousness is a dangerous thing, as Icarus discovered when his waxen wings melted in the glare of the Sun.

To stick a flag on the surface of the Moon is to announce conquest. Conquest is interference. The Moon gives us the rhythm of life through the tides and the menstrual cycle. The conquest of the Moon took place at the same time as stringent birth control measures were in practice throughout the world: in the 'undeveloped' world sterilisation was promoted while in the 'developed' world all kinds of contraception was suddenly available. The sixties generation of young women who were the first imbibers of the

Pill has now graduated. Those lucky ladies, accustomed to taking their little pill each day to affect radically the hormone balance of their bodies are now on more daily doses: Hormone Replacement Treatment keeps their bodies as artificially imbalanced as ever. Meanwhile, the incidence of cancers attacking the female organs has reached alarming proportions.

The rhythms of our bodies and minds are inseparable from the motions of the planets of the solar system as they wind their way through the universe. It is pointless to talk of the necessity of recreating a link with our environment unless we also become aware of the rhythms of the universe. Our environment is not only the landscape around us; it is the interconnectedness of the planetary system we are part of, and of all that lies within and beyond it.

Meditation exercise
to link the centre of the head with the lower part of the body.

Sit comfortably with the spine as straight as possible.

Bring your awareness to the base of the spine, or coccyx. Try to make a good contact - it can be quite difficult to find.

With your awareness, move up the spine, up the cervical spine in the neck and from there into the centre of the head.

Pause there and allow any sensation to take place.

Travel back down the spine to the coccyx and pause there.

Continue to move up and down between the coccyx and the centre of the head, pausing at each place, and finish, after ten minutes or so, at the coccyx.

Two

The Moon   The Pituitary

'We look not at the things which are seen, but at the things which are not seen: for the things which are seen are temporal, but the things which are not seen are eternal.'

2 Corinthians 4;18

The nursery rhymes of my childhood led me to believe that, while little boys were made of slugs and snails and puppy dogs' tails, little girls, like me, were made of sugar and spice and all things nice. Little boys were horrid, violent creatures like Georgie Porgie. They pulled the wings off butterflies and chased us little girls when all we wanted to do was to arrange our cockle shells and silver bells, eat our curds and whey and lead our pet lambs to school.

It came as something of a shock, then, to learn that I had got it all wrong. The truth of the matter was that boys were good and girls were bad. Everyone in the know said so: priests, rabbis, ayatollahs, Zen masters, bishops, sages - and God himself. Girls, in fact, were evil and that is why they were not allowed to sing in the church choir or play football in the school playground. When they grew up they were given permission to make the cucumber sandwiches and wash the rugby kit and were allowed to arrange the flowers in the church and drop their savings into the collecting tin, but God forbid they take over the scoring, the umpiring, the law-making or the preaching.

When I used to tell the boys in the school playground that they were slimy and smelly they usually had an answer and didn't hesitate to give it. But there was no arguing with the Church. It wasn't men who had made up the rules, it was God. It just so happened that God had said that not only were women unclean, they were also unable to communicate directly with God. This meant that women were dependent on men to tell them who they were and where they belonged. Men, on the whole, seemed quite happy to perform this task. And, luckily, men had the great advantage over women of objectivity. They could hear the God-given truth and pass it on unaffected by emotional considerations.

Countless men have been (and still are) persecuted for querying the tenets of orthodox religion. The history of the world is the history of religious persecution. But women have been (and still are) persecuted not only for questioning religious doctrines but for being women: for expressing womanly thoughts or for behaving in womanly ways.

Women have been required, throughout patriarchal societies, to obey their husbands since their husbands carry the will of God. And all kinds of devices and laws have been created to ensure they do, from total economic dependence to the scold's bridle (a harness worn over the head with a sharp metal point digging into the mouth), to bound feet, clitoredectomies and to the 'rule of thumb' (an English law that gave men permission to beat their wives with a stick no thicker than their thumb). In some Arab societies today, old men congregate in shopping malls and markets and hit women's ankles with sticks if they are considered to have transgressed the strict dress code.

> "A woman, a dog, a walnut tree,
> The more you beat them, the better they'll be."

Males and females both oppress and suffer oppression, slavery exists across the board. But, in religious thinking, female and black are associated with negative, with the Devil, and are incapable of rising above their base natures. And, because male and white have God on their side, they can do nothing wrong.

The concept of polarity resides in every system of thought. It suggests that everything is in flux, in the process, of changing into its opposite. Day becomes night and the first becomes last. But political systems and established religions are incapable of adaptation and flexibility, religious thought tends to harden into unarguable doctrine, and the profound philosophy of polarity has rigidified throughout the world into a system of opposites based on a sense of superiority and inferiority which justifies oppression (although why it should be just for the strong to oppress the weak is another matter).

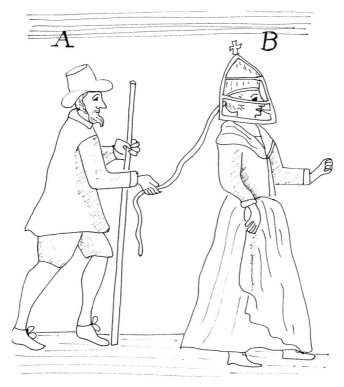

The scold's bridle. England. 18th century.

Black and negative are associated with the female while white and positive are identified with the male. Anyone who has had to fill in any kind of Government form will also know that M belongs with number 1 and F with number 2. In all my years of applying for driving licences, child benefit, passports, school dinners and other necessities of our civilisation, I have never been promoted to number 1.

Two, of course, is secondary to number one. It is a follower, a shadow, an echo. It is easily overlooked although to ignore it may be one's own undoing. As it was for Narcissus. On the day he sat brooding on his own reflection, his own iris, he was being watched. One of the numerous nymphs who were in love with the beautiful boy was Echo and the day of Narcissus's untimely death she had followed him and was lurking in the woods waiting for him to notice her. Drugged on his own fascinating image, he was too absorbed to take his eyes away from himself but if he had, he would have been saved.

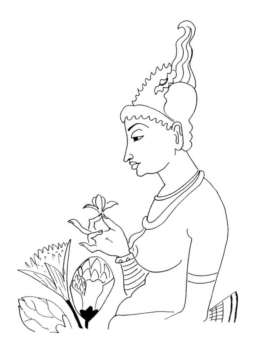

Nymph with lily or lotus. Tibet. 5th century.

A 'nymph' is a beautiful young woman and the *nympha* are the external female genital organs: the clitoris and inner labia. Nympha also means 'a white and yellow lily'. The inner labia are contained within the outer, called in Sanskrit the *yoni* and in Latin, the *vesica*, a pointed oval shape associated with the Virgin Mary who is also identified with the lily.

If Narcissus had pulled his sight away from his own iris and looked instead at Echo, number two, he would have found the nymph, the lily, the sexual parts that would have received his own and created a whole, a boat, a container, a vessel to save him from drowning in his own small pool.

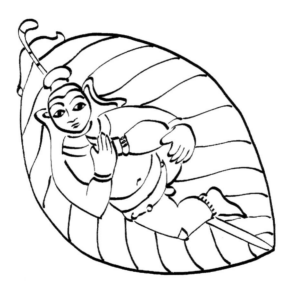

The god, Krishna, on a vesica-shaped leaf. India. 19th century.

There was little that the neglected Echo could do to save Narcissus, condemned as she was only to reflect and respond, never to initiate. Number two has no light of its own but, like the Moon to the Sun, merely reflects the light of number one. In English speaking societies the female is associated with the Moon and the Moon is considered of secondary importance to the Sun. Silver, the reflection, is worth less than gold, the true substance. And, not only is the Moon less substantial than the Sun, she is also fickle and unpredictable. While the steady old Sun consistently does his thing, shining out with all his might to keep us going, the irresponsible Moon flirts and hides, is devious and unstable, swinging from one mood to another.

The orbit of Earth and Moon around the Sun is what makes our calendar and our clock. The spin of Earth creates the day, our rotation round the Sun creates the year and the seasons and the Moon's movements in relation to both Earth and Sun make the months and weeks. It seems that pre-patriarchal cultures described the Moon as leading the path through the heavens that the Sun followed but patriarchal cultures see the Sun as leader and Moon as follower.

A calendar is a ruler, regulating time through the observation of the movements of heavenly bodies. In French the word for ruler is *la regle* and its plural, *les regles* means menstrual periods. Both the English and French colloquialisms for menstruation link it with the regulation of time and the word 'menstruation' itself comes from 'menses', meaning measurement.

While the Sun can be identified with light and fire, the Moon is associated with darkness and water. The Sun, number one, provides the sense of a separate identity but the Moon, governing the ebbs and flows, the tides of life, links one being to another. Women who live together tend to ovulate and menstruate at the same time. Our way of living as separate couples has divided women from each other and our recent tendency to encourage husbands or male partners to take over the traditional roles of supportive females in pregnancy, childbirth and childcare brings the danger of isolating women still further from each other (as well as making nervous wrecks of our menfolk).

The menstrual cycle has obvious connections with the phases of the Moon and with the tides. Many women experience either ovulation or menstruation at full Moon and, therefore, the opposite polarity at the dying Moon. Having kept records of my own cycle over many years, I discovered that ovulation and full Moon occurred more or less concurrently for a good many months and then, over a duration of two or three months, would adjust to the other polarity and stay there for a length of time before changing back. The influence of the Moon and the tides is a collective one, affecting

L V N A .

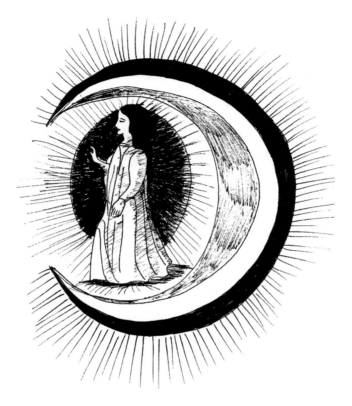

Luna, the Roman goddess of the Moon. 15th century

us en masse. Our lives and our fates are interrelated, like the weavings of a web. When women lived together in the sacred, private thalamus their power was inseparable from the times and the tides, the menses. The regular monthly motion of growth towards ovulation and fertility and the decline into the dissolution and shedding of menstruation is reflected in the waxing and waning of the Moon and the ebb and flow of the tides. The rhythm of life, the weavings of destiny, were centred in the women's room or thalamus.

The way we live now in the developed world has, through separating women from each other, affected the rhythms not only of individual women but of society. Countless women suffer from irregular and painful menstrual cycles, taking no end of substances and even operations to try to 'cure' the problem. But the problem lies in their isolation. The menstrual cycle is not meant to be a lonely secretive affair and neither can it be set right by the lone woman. We are, by nature, tribal beings and in most mammalian societies females and their offspring live together while the males live the more solitary life, attaching themselves from time to time to a group.

The regulator of the menstrual cycle and the chief endocrine gland is the pituitary gland in the centre of the head. So it can be assumed that the pituitary has a relationship to the Moon. While the pineal, 'the seat of the soul', has links with the Sun, giving us our orientation in time and space and our sense of day and night, the pituitary, by giving authority to the other glands to secrete their hormones, makes it possible for us to function; to sleep, wake, think, talk, digest, excrete, make love, reproduce and so on.

The pineal governs the upward moving, 'masculine' elements of fire and air, while the pituitary governs the downward moving, 'feminine' elements of earth and water. 'Pituitary' means 'slime' and slime is, of course, a mixture of earth and water, the mud or clay from which, in many myths, we were originally formed. Fire and air belong to soul and spirit; earth and water to matter and emotion. In countless philosophies, fire and air are the substance of the Father while water and earth belong to the Mother.

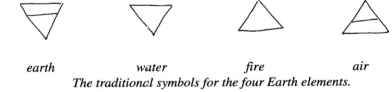

| earth | water | fire | air |

The traditional symbols for the four Earth elements.

Latin for mother is *mater* from which arise 'mate', 'matter', material' and 'mattress'. The mother and the Earth form the matrix, the very fabric of life, and yet the value accorded to both mothers and the Earth has been so diminished that plenty of mothers might also relate to another associated word: 'doormat'.

Dumping waste in the earth, rivers and seas is, as the Amerindians warned time and again, akin to polluting one's own family. But now, not only have we left graffiti on even the most sacred mountain peaks, altered the very structure of the rivers and seas with our chemicals, and exploded nuclear bombs beneath the surface of the earth but, like spoiled children waiting for some mother-drudge to tidy up behind us, we leave our discarded toys in space as well.

We have so upset the natural balance that we no longer have a sense of women at the heart of society. If we speak of society having a 'heart' we are usually referring to the banking or political centres. The thalamus is no longer honoured, the source has been forgotten. Women throughout the world are treated more or less as slaves (it is estimated that women own 2% of the world's wealth) and our seas, lakes, rivers and all things that depend on water are dying. As long as money-making and not child-rearing is seen as the heart of society, the Earth, the seas, the sky and even space itself will continue to be exploited and abused. Leaving technological litter in space and dumping nuclear waste in the seas is tantamount to defecating in your living room with the important difference that no Mrs Mop can take her scrubbing brush and clean it up.

The material world is our mother, providing us with the Earth and the nourishment we need to survive but the Mother is also the sea and the source, the waters of the deep. Water is fundamental: it accounts for 70% of our bodies and of the Earth's surface. It was in water that the origins of life were formed. Our bodies, like the Earth, contain a mixture of clear and salt water: while our saliva is akin to clear spring water, our blood, sweat and tears are salt as is the albumen, the fluid that contains the baby in the womb. Albumen, meaning simply, 'white', refers to both the white of an egg and the white of the eye; it is the watery substance that contains and nourishes the incarnating soul. Water is highly sensitive and a super-swift conductor of energy, that is to say, of the radiation of the Sun. The very fine water of the Earth's atmosphere channels and filters the Sun's rays to make them acceptable to life. Water cleanses and carries away waste but is deeply affected by pollution.

French for mother is 'la mere' which is pronounced the same as the word for the sea, 'la mer'. Related to it is the English 'mare', the female horse said by the Greeks to turn her hindquarters to the North wind since that is where the seed comes from that impregnates all females. (The male sea-

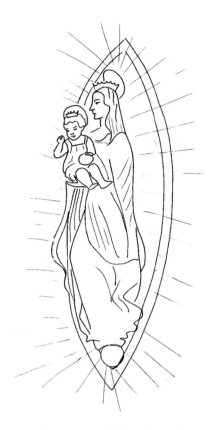

Virgin and child in the vesica

horse, incidentally, is the only male of any species to become pregnant.) The Great Mere, Mer, Mare or Mother is, of course, Mary who is identified with both the blue of heaven and of the sea and is sometimes depicted as a Moon Goddess. Her symbol is the vesica piscis, or fish vessel, a yoni or vulva shape that surrounds spiritual beings and is also known as a mandorla (meaning almond), the counterpart to the circular, solar, male mandala. It is created from two overlapping circles.

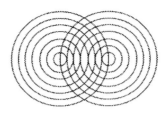

When those interpenetrating circles themselves form other circles, as in the formation of a tree trunk or by casting a stone into still water, many vesicas (or waves) are formed. Leonardo da Vinci observed this motion:

'If you throw two stones at the same time on to a sheet of motionless water at some distance from one another, you will see that around the two percussions two quantities of separate circles are caused, which as they increase in size will meet and then penetrate and intersect one another, whilst all the time maintaining as their respective centres the places percussed by the stones'.

After the death of her son, known by gnostic Christians as the Fish, Mary is said to have sailed the Mediterranean to the South of France. All along the French coast are reminders of her arrival with Mary Magdalen and Mary Jacobin and their subsequent inhabitance of the region. Time and again, groups of three women are found in mythology. They relate to the phases of the Moon and of Venus, they are the Fates, the Graces and the Triple Goddess, ordering our lives, regulating time and destiny.

Three mothers contain, determine and protect our consciousness, existing not only as archetypes beyond us but as entities within us. They are found surrounding our brains and spinal columns, three protective membranes, known as the pia mater, the arachnoid mater and the dura mater: the young and slender mother, the spider mother and the hard mother or crone. Spinal, or cerebral, fluid, the salt water located in the ventricles, is constantly drawn to the three membranes where it circulates the cerebro/spinal system and, through the arachnoid mater, is spread into the brain by means of little spidery villi or rivulets.

The pool of water in the centre of the head, constantly refreshed and revitalised, the never-ending source, is situated between the pineal and pituitary glands and is known as the third ventricle which extends into the

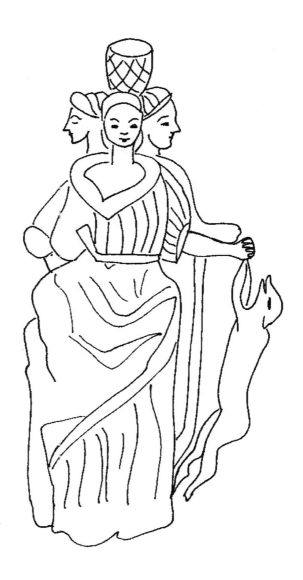

Hecate, the Greek triple goddess of the Moon.

thalamus. The thalamus has been described as the size and shape of a small hen's egg. Thalamus also means: 'sacred space', 'temple of the bee', 'receptacle of the flower' (the container that holds the seeds, for instance, the entire flesh or fruit of an apple or strawberrry that is left after the flower has dropped), and 'women's room'. If the foetal-shaped brain, surrounded by its three nourishing and protective mothers, had a navel, it would be situated so that its umbilical cord would be attached to the thalamus.

Together, the conscious brain and the thalamus are child and mother, male and female. They are the combination of the solar principle of consciousness or oneness, symbolised by the dot within the circle and of the lunar principle of the subconscious, the supportive linking waters, symbolised by the vesica. When the circle of the Sun is located within the vesica of the Moon, when Narcissus, the iris, enters the nympha or inner labia, conception can occur and the soul can incarnate in its body surrounded by its aura (its breath or spirit), Echo offers Narcissus a ship on which to voyage the sea of life and the union of one and two bring into being the number three, the third or single eye.

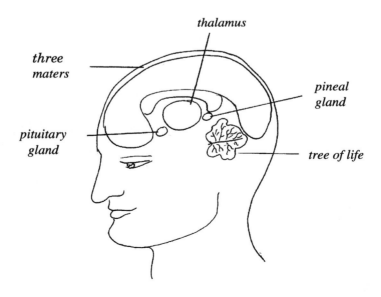

An exercise

This exercise is to relate the energy of the lower part of the body with the energy of the head. Exercises like this one have been performed over the centuries in monasteries. In such exercises, energy is drawn up the body from the perineum point. The perineum point is situated between the testicles and the anus in men and between the vagina and the anus in women. But, in women, the G-spot, a point on the front wall of the vagina, is much stronger than the perineum point so it is better for women to draw energy up from the G-spot.

Sit comfortably.

Bring your awareness to the perineum point or G-spot.

Rest there.

Then come up the front of the spine, following it up through the neck, into the centre of the head.

Rest in the centre of the head.

Return down the front of the spine to the perineum point or G-spot and rest.

Repeat the movement up and down for ten minutes or so, finishing at the perineum point or G-spot.

Three
Mercury   The Thyroid

'You can't make an omelette without breaking eggs.'

Old saying

The universe, some myths tell us, was hatched from the cosmic egg. Like the eye, the egg is a symbol of the union of male and female. Not only is the fertilised egg the result of the union of those two fundamental forces but its form represents them, the golden yolk being the image of the Sun and consciousness and the silvery white or albumen belonging to the waters of the Moon, the unconscious.

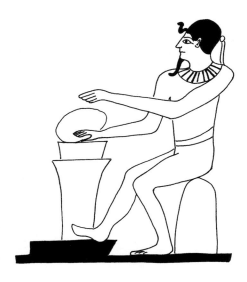

The Egyptian god, Ptah, fashioning the cosmic egg

The cosmic egg was laid by the dove of innocence and hatched by the snake of experience which coiled round the egg seven times so splitting it into seven parts or levels. Seven forms the scale: of the inner planets, the chakras, the colours, the musical notes, and of the days of the week which themselves are created by the monthly dance of Sun and Moon. The whole of creation is released in the hatching of the egg and is the result of the union of the male and female forces of light and water, consciousness and the unconscious.

In the centre of our heads, beneath the cerebral cortex, lies the thalamus. Scientists suggest that, while the thalamus does not in itself contain consciousness, it acts as a central exchange. It is, some say, like a torch, shining onto the part of the brain that is in use at that moment, which then, through its dependency on the thalamus, becomes the seat of consciousness.

The Bible tells us that through the action of sound and light, God created the world and all that is in it. But that creation, like the Big Bang, did not only happen once. It is a continual process. Creation is infinite and perpetual. The light of God's eye shining on the void, the waters of the deep, creates a massive reflection. Reflection is, therefore, creation and creation is born of the eye of consciousness. The thalamus (echoing the Greek for 'sea', *thalassa*) and the deep well of the third ventricle could be said to be the source of all things.

It is possible to link each part of the creation story to the make-up of the brain. At the back of the brain lies the cerebellum, also known as the tree of life and either side of the thalamus lies a snake, the cauda (a Latin word meaning tail). The snake, of course, is responsible for the Fall. Through the temptation of the snake, we have descended from Paradise to the suffering state of humanity. In hatching the cosmic egg, the snake brought the inspiration of God into manifestation. It is responsible for bringing to birth everything in creation but is also guilty of breakage, having caused the initial fragmentation from unity. But without the action of the snake, the egg can have no experience or development. The snake is essential to growth, to knowledge and to the struggle for union between the sexes. From the union of male and female, one and two, comes the number three.

'The Tao begot one.
One begot two.

Two begot three.
And three begot the ten thousand things,'

says Lao Tsu, the ancient Chinese philosopher.

Three is the child produced from the union of sperm and ovum, the creative life force that comes from the marriage of Sun and Moon. One is gold, two is silver, three is copper, the element that, because of its ability to carry energy at great speed, is used, coiled, to conduct electricity and forms the basis of lightning conductors. Copper earths energy and the snake, by bringing down the energy of Sun and Moon, enables that energy to manifest as all of creation, what the Chinese call 'the ten thousand things'.

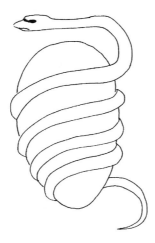

Alchemical image

The movement of energy in the human being is closely associated with the movement of spinal fluid, the light salt water that circulates the brain and spins up and down the spine, forming the central nervous system which links the nerves of the whole body to the brain. The word 'spin' is related to the word 'spine' and the word 'vertebra' means 'to turn'. The motion of energy in the spinal cord is a spiral.

The spine is what separates the individual from the mass. Creatures of the Earth are divided into two sorts: vertebrates and invertebrates. And with the physical classification go innumerable symbolic implications. Invertebrates belong to the mass: they have no will, decisiveness or individuality. But those who have backbone have strength, determination and ambition. While the spineless suffer from fear, timidity and lack of conviction, those with a spine are dignified and courageous.

Even among the majestic family of independent and motivated vertebrates, man is special. The spine of man is vertical. He is upright, conscious and proud. His spine is the sword of truth and justice. It is the symbol of the integrity of the individual and, when it is constructed as column, totem pole or post, it is the structure that proclaims the values of nations, families, cultures and civilisations.

When Samson was seduced by Delilah of the Philistines and robbed of his hair, symbol of spiritual and sexual potency, and, therefore, stripped of his physical strength, he managed as his final act to push down the pillars of the grand hall of the Philistines and destroy the house of the beliefs of his enemy. Perhaps the influence of a civilisation has not entirely waned until its last pillar has crumbled. Samson is the prime example of mind overcoming matter. Though his emotions were seduced, his spirit regained its strength.

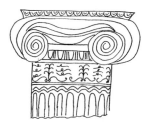

The spine is the link between head and body or thought and physical response. Like copper, it carries energy to Earth. And that energy itself can be compared to quicksilver. Quicksilver or mercury is used in thermometers to measure the distribution and regulation of heat and in instruments to measure blood pressure and atmospheric conditions. It is tremendously sensitive to heat while not in itself being affected by it. If you place some

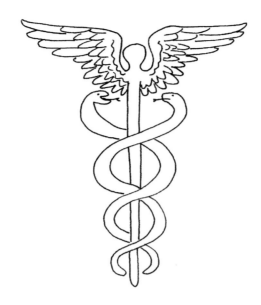

The caduceus

mercury on a plate or tray and give it only the tiniest movement, it speeds across the surface like a very intelligent silverfish defying you to believe it is not alive. Though it may break and divide, it joins together again as if it had never been separated. Mercury is the smallest planet and, although it is comparatively near the Earth, it is almost invisible, partly because it is so small but chiefly because it is so near the Sun that it is lost in the Sun's rays.

Mercury is the little fleet messenger of the Sun, linking mortals with the gods and the gods with the source. He wears a helmet to protect him from the Sun and make him invisible and wings on his ankles. His instrument is the flute, made from the reed which grows in water and is, like the spine, sectioned into vertebrae. Mercury catches the divine breath and from it makes harmony and melody. He is the child of Jove (Jupiter or Zeus), king of the gods and has much in common with Christ who also was the son of God and, born of a virgin or nymph, remained of the spirit, descending to Earth with a message and with healing powers.

Mercury's healing powers are located in his wand, known as the caduceus up which weave two snakes, their heads usually depicted facing each other at the top.

These are snakes of solar and lunar energies that Mercury carries up the spine with its seven chakras which, as they spin, draw energy in and sends it out. The chakras, in turn, each relate to one of the glands which release hormones into the blood, enabling the body to function. So the spine not only gauges the temperature or emotional field of the whole system, it also links the brain to the circulation of the nervous system and to the circulation of the blood.

The two snakes of Mercury are an age-old representation of the energies that modern science locates in the image of the double helix ('helix' means 'coil' or 'spiral' and 'helios' is the Sun). The double helix carries the DNA or genetic structure from the original gene pool through the individuals of each generation and therefore represents continuity in time.

The fundamental formation of time - which we see in the clock and the calendar - stems from the motions of the Sun and Moon in relation to the Earth, in other words, from the pineal, or inner sundial, and the pituitary, or inner regulator, in relation to our own bodies.

The original source or gene pool is the void, the waters of the deep. If the heads of the solar and lunar snakes of the caduceus can be seen as the pineal and pituitary then the bowl-like space created between their two necks is the thalamus. The word 'thalamus' refers not only to the space in the centre of the head from which consciousness arises, not only to the women's room from which all life is born, but to the receptacle of a flower, containing all the seeds for the future; and the spine of the flower is its stalk.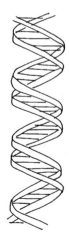

The double helix, like the twisting snakes, forms a spiral of entwining energies which are held together by a series of rungs so the whole structure looks like a spiralling ladder. In the caduceus the rungs are the meeting places of the twisting serpents and mark the positions of the chakras. The snakes and the double helix look something like a plait. But a plait, though it appears to be constructed of two entwining locks, is actually formed from three, the third being the invisible force or spirit that gives the two the strength to bind together. The two snakes of the caduceus wind themselves up a rod or wand, which is sometimes depicted and sometimes invisible. This is the magic wand, the healing or divining rod of Mercury. It is the very essence of the spinal column. And Mercury is the invisible spirit who, like Cupid, Puck or Ariel, can bring together disparate forces for good or bad.

Snakes carry the power of healing and of poison and the two words in Greek are almost the same: *pharmakia* means poison and *pharmakion*, healing. Mercury can have a seriously detrimental effect on the central nervous system but he is also the divine messenger and healer and, when tamed and controlled, his power is immense. Until recently, mercury was the only remedy for syphilis, prompting the wry saying that 'a night with Venus leads to a lifetime with Mercury'.

Though the spine can be associated with righteousness and truth, Mercury is also the divine trickster, a thief and a liar. His messages may be twisted and devious and lead to the misuse of energy. All illness, it has been said, is a resistance to truth and the spinal fluid carries within it all memories of truth and deceit. Man may have fallen through heeding the appeal of the snake, but it is through the snake that he ascends again. He can never recapture the state of innocence, but, through experience, he can attain wisdom and healing.

Mercury provides the binding force for the powers of male and female, Sun and Moon to meet. He is the child that holds the parents together, the cherub that entices them to procreation. His invisible force creates the seven levels, the ladder between heaven and Earth. These are the levels of manifestation and each one is identified with a chakra. If the Sun and Moon can be located in the head and linked to the pineal chakra (encompassing both the pineal and pituitary glands), then Mercury, the messenger who forms a bridge between Father/pineal, Mother/pituitary, and the other chakras/planets, can be identified with the thyroid chakra in the neck.

The neck is a bridge between head and body, with its own mini-spine of seven cervical vertebrae. 'Cervix' means opening and 'thyroid' means gateway. Mercury provides the meeting place: between the gods and humans and between the female and the male. In Greece Mercury was known as Hermes and in Egypt as Hermes Trismegistus, the 'thrice-risen'.

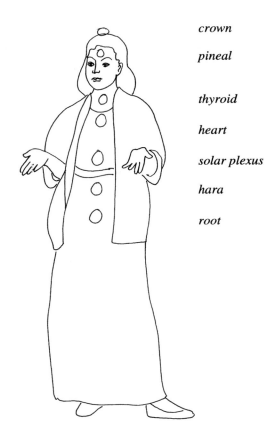

crown

pineal

thyroid

heart

solar plexus

hara

root

As the link between heaven and Earth, his temples were often built on hill-tops. Many still stand, dedicated, like St. Michael's Mount and Mont St. Michel, to the Archangel Michael whose powers of intervention between humanity and the gods overlap with those of Mercury.

In releasing the seven levels of energy, Mercury creates the ladder of the rainbow, enabling Iris to spiral down with her paintpot and paint each chakra a different colour. Reflecting an interesting mish-mash of cultures, the names we use for the chakras are a mixture of Latin, Greek, English and Sanskrit. To the pineal, Iris gives indigo, to the thyroid sky blue, green to the heart and yellow to the solar plexus while the hara (a Sanskrit word meaning 'soul') gets orange and the root, red. In this way she descends

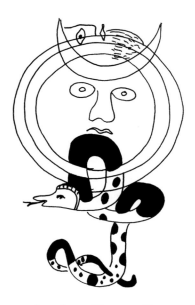

Sun, Moon and snake or Mercury. Europe. 16th century.

through her rainbow in order saving the final, highest frequency colour, violet, for the crown above the head.

The rainbow is the covenant between God and man formed after the Great Flood. It is a symbol of order, a message from God to affirm that there is, after all, meaning and purpose to life. Our origins may be dark and watery but the action of light on water gives us the hierarchy of colour and tone, the ladder on which to find our way up and down between thought and emotion and between spirit and matter with awareness and harmony.

Mercury, as the messenger, carries the word. It is through him we can communicate and through him that the word can be put into practice. His feathers not only allow him to speed between the light of thought and the human organs of speech, but can be used as quills with which to write. He enables all forms of communication and, through the thyroid chakra, opens our ears and mouths.

The thyroid chakra, like the gland, has three parts, the two outer circles dependent on the central one, just as the two outer lobes of the gland are linked by the large central one, known as the pyramidial lobe and having that shape.

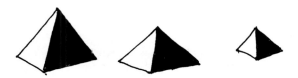

The pyramids of Abu Sir, Eygpt.

The pyramids were constructed as meeting places between the gods and humanity, places to mark the passage, the gateway between life and death, between mortal form and immortal soul. Their shafts, pointing to specific celestial bodies, seem to have allowed the souls of dead kings to return to their homes in the stars.

The pyramid descends from a unified point to a square plane through the medium of the triangle. Mercury, creating the link between left and right, female and male, forms the stability, the balance and the healing power of the triangle, and, as the third party to the trinity, he is the angel, spirit or dove carrying messages of peace and goodwill. He is both the snake that hatched the cosmic egg and the dove that laid it, both the snake that takes us crashing down to Earth and the ladder that gives us the opportunity to make our way back to heaven.

A meditation

Imagine a light blue colour above your head.

Let the colour drop all round you as if forming an egg shape, bringing it down beneath your feet.

Repeat this several times until you feel you have made a good contact with the colour.

If you can't contact the colour, never mind. Just thinking of the word 'blue' will have an effect.

Then let go of the colour and bring your awareness to either of these words: 'peace or silence'.

Let your thoughts go where they will.

At the end of a fifteen minute period, or when you feel ready, bring light up from beneath the feet to above the head, forming an egg-shape.

(The same meditation can be done another time using the colour pink and one of the words, 'sharing' or 'giving'; or with the colour gold and the word 'attraction' or 'protection'.)

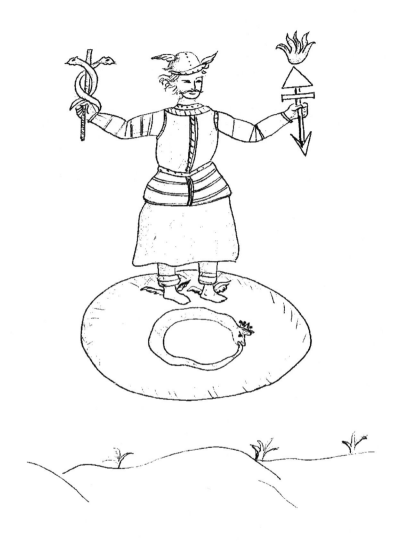

Mercury on the egg, the shape of the planet's orbit. Inside it, as yolk, is the ouroborous, the snake that swallows its own tail. Europe. 17th century.

Four

Venus and the Earth   The Heart

'All things do live in the three; but in the four they merry be'.
Alchemical saying

The dove, like the lily, is a symbol of purity and innocence and the snake, like the red rose, is one of experience. Life on Earth is about experience. You can't make an omelette without breaking eggs and you can't have the richness of mortal life without the snake hatching the egg of innocence.

It is, of course, woman who is first tempted by the snake. In Christianity, woman is Eve; in the Roman pantheon which still informs the astronomical/astrological system used in the west today, woman is Venus. In the Bible stories of the life of Jesus, women are scarce. There are no female disciples and the two women close to Jesus are his mother, the Virgin, and the Magdalene, the ex-prostitute. Similarly, in Roman astrology, there are only two goddesses: the Moon, or Virgin and Mother, and Venus, the full-bloodied sexual temptress. There is no more point in looking for complexity of character in these female archetypes than there is in making an in-depth psychological analysis of Minnie Mouse.

Femaleness in cartoons is represented by an apron (mother) or by fluttering eyelashes (whore). Cartoons, like most literature and art, are about males relating to each other. Tom has Jerry, Bill has Ben, Batman has Robin, Noddy has Big Ears, Robin Hood has his band of Merrie Men, King Arthur has a whole court of knights and Jesus has a dozen disciples. The male group, like the signs of the zodiac, gives expression to the different aspects of the psyche and provides the opportunity for an understanding and exploration of how these aspects relate to each other. In some stories this purpose is quite clear - each of the Seven Dwarfs, for instance, has the name of a human characteristic: Sleepy, Grumpy and so on.

50

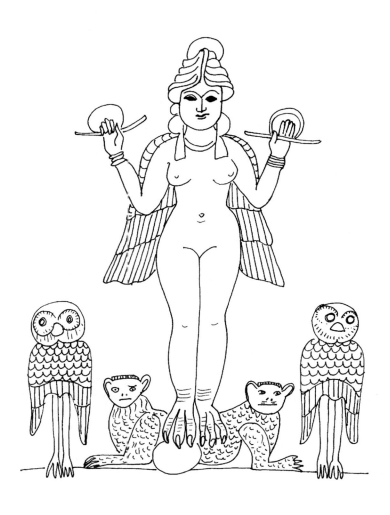

Lilith. Sumer. C 2,000 B.C.

The female, when she appears at all, is without character. She is simply Good or Bad, Snow White or the wicked Queen. Either she fits the tradition of Cinderella, the Virgin Mary, Little Weed, Maid Marian and assorted anonymous princesses in towers or she is a baddie like the first woman, Lilith, who was so wicked she had to be banished from the face of the Earth to be superseded by the marginally less evil but gullible Eve and countless other dumb, cruel and jealous types like Pandora, Delilah, Morgana le Fay, Cruella de Ville and a range of ugly stepmothers and sisters.

Good and bad are white and red or innocence and experience. Women are either lilies or roses. And while the Moon may be associated with the lily and the Virgin, Venus is woman as flesh and blood, sexual, carnal and sinful.

Just as the name Eve echoes the word evil so the name of Venus has its links with sin, poison and blood. 'Venus venerari' means sexual love and from the same root comes 'venal'. A venal sin in Catholicism is one that must be pardoned since it cannot be avoided. Simply by being incarnated in flesh we have sinned, tempted by the snake through its seductive and poisonous speech, its 'venom'. Like the snake, Venus and Eve entice but what they promise is unreal and deadly.

Venus was born of the union of heaven and the sea, conceived when the testicles of Uranos, the god of heaven, were cut off and thrown into the ocean. She emerged from a scallop surrounded by mists. It is the mist itself, the action of the seed of Uranos on the sea, or the eye of God on the void, that brings humanity into being. Mist or steam arises when light or heat meets cold water. The effect of God's voice on the frozen waters of the deep was to crack the ice and the action of the light that he summonsed was to melt it. From the combined powers of God's voice - sound - and the look of his eye - light - the cosmos was born. Conception occurs through the medium of sound. It is sound that attracts the sperm to the ovum. Sound and hearing precede light and seeing - as we know from thunderstorms and from waiting for underground trains. But light brings life into being. In numerous religions, life is said to be illusion, woven by the spider and formed of mist and steam. All that we reach for is false; we are locked in the wheel of confusion, chasing phantasms.

The state of illusion, the veil, is known as the goddess Maya, a word that echoes 'maioid', Greek for sea-spider. The maioid, or arachnoid mater,

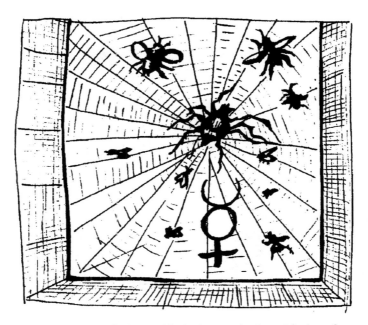

Mercury is trapped along with the insects in the spider's web.
Alchemical image.

distributes salt water through the brain, feeding and nourishing
consciousness. Another Greek name for the sea-spider is 'nymphon'; and a
nymphon is also a bridal chamber. Traditionally, the nymphon adjoined the
women's quarters of the House, the thalamus. (The thalamus, of course,
does not belong to the house of the nuclear family - it is the inner centre of
the House and the House is not only a large building complete with
courtyards and other dwellings, but is the community itself with its
hierarchy organised around the ruling family). Men could not enter the
thalamus and could go no further than the nymphon whose relation to the
inner sanctum was a social and architectural replica of the vagina's relation
to the womb.

As bridal chamber, the nymphon was a place of great beauty and sensuality,
ruled over by the god Hymen who is normally depicted as a young man
carrying a torch and a veil and who gives his name to the 'hymenoptera', a
group of winged insects that includes wasps and bees. In Greece you can

53

still see the old ladies making lace bedspreads for the nuptials and in India lavish decorations are prepared for the wedding chamber. All over the world, the bride is still enveloped in veils, silks and lace. She is the embodiment of Maya, an incarnation of Venus. Shrouded in the mists of illusion, she is, like Earthly life itself, full of promise, enticing and mysterious and yet only temporal, doomed to disappoint and die. Venus, sexual and mortal, contains within her the seeds of death. Pure, white and virginal though the bride may seem, she is really made of flesh and blood and blood is the stuff of suffering and sacrifice.

Venus has many sisters but, unlike the Merrie Men, dwarfs, disciples or knights, they have no Earthly identity. They are simply the Furies. When Venus emerged as the first sex object, the Furies sank as drops of blood to the bottom of the ocean. They are the waste, the menstrual blood that does not go towards conception and the formation of new life. Not a direct part of the heritage of life, they are also known as the Fates, condemned to mutter their curses from outside society, from below the surface of consciousness.

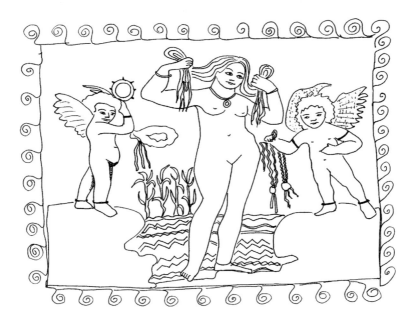

Venus. Mosaic from Tunisia

Venus, unlike the Virgin who, some claim, came herself from a virgin birth, was conceived of a full union of male (heaven) and female (the sea). Emerging from the fertilised egg, she is the pearl of conception and the mother of life. She is the child of experience, of the sea of humanity, represented by blood.

Venus and blood share the same name. 'Venous' blood is blood that is spent, returning through the veins to the heart, depleted of air. Blood without air can be likened to emotion without reason and diseases of the blood may often be related to unconscious emotion. Diabetes, for instance, seems to have a connection to jealousy while anaemia can be traced to fear and inhibition. Jaundice, a condition of the blood that can be cured by exposure to light, has given its name to a state of mind that is negative and tired.

Wicked queens who pass their days asking vain questions of their mirrors and plotting jealous acts of wrath against young nymphs suffer from diseases of the blood. In time, their beautiful faces turn 'green and pale'. Blood that does not have access to air, light or reason is the blood of the vampire. The vampire feeds on blood, loves the dark, is addicted to the flesh, seeks to corrupt young innocents with blood-lust and appears to have no conscience, no higher mind. It is a creature of night, akin to the bat and, of course, to the witch.

Despite the vampire's inordinate power of destruction, there are ways to restrain him. Expose him to the light, stay his approach by displaying a cross, protect yourself with garlic and, if you can, kill him by driving a stake though his heart.

To control the power of the vampire is to control one's own unconscious desires. The methods used in vampire taming can be applied to oneself: to expose the vampire to the light is to subject one's passions to the light of consciousness and reason; displaying the cross can be interpreted as developing faith; garlic is renowned for its ability to purify the blood, which, symbolically, is the purification of experience or the release from the power of the past. The ultimate achievement of freedom from the dominance of the passions is by putting a stake through the heart which is to put the heart to rest by rising above all sensory desire.

The vampire belongs to the darkness and the unconscious and has a strong relationship to the devil. It is a creature of the two lower elements, earth and water. Air and fire, the elements of light, are antithetical to its nature. It lives on blood but the blood of the vampire is without air; it is venous blood.

Blood represents both the experience of the individual and the sharing of humanity. In the Christian church the partaking of the wine symbolises the individual's willingness to share in the sufferings of Christ and, through him, of mankind. It gives the means for redemption from the agony of the cross. But blood may also symbolise division, into families, nations and races. We develop blood ties, engage in blood feuds and cause blood baths. 'Vengeance', with its companion words - revenge, avenge, vendetta - also comes from the same root as 'venal'. Through blood we experience and suffer but, also through the blood, we reach atonement, forgiveness and redemption.

> *'Teach me to repent, for that's as good*
> *As if thou hadst sealed my pardon with thy blood.'* - John Donne

Myths tell us that humanity has fallen from grace and that we are guilty of original sin. Sexual desire, it would seem, is our undoing. Though the word venal may have its links with poison, sin and vengeance, it also gives rise to 'venia' which means 'forgiveness' and 'venerari', meaning 'veneration'. Worship and atonement are as much a part of being human as is sexual desire and it can be through sexual love ('venus venerari') that we develop a sense of awe, respect and veneration.

Venus is the goddess of sexuality and, therefore, mortality but she is also goddess of love, harmony and peace. During the long period of world-wide patriarchal religion that is only now drawing to an end crude religious and cultural doctrine and practice has taken the easy option of positing woman as the accomplice of the devil, occupied only with matters of the body and the emotions. Man, correspondingly, has been seen as of the spirit, aligned with God and charged with the task of subduing nature, of which woman has been seen as part.

The symbol for Venus, though taken up by feminists as representing womanhood, is akin to the Egyptian ankh, the symbol of life.

It is a stick-man, a head over a body shown by the circle of spirit over the cross of matter. We are all of woman and of Venus born, we are all spirits in mortal bodies, we are all stick-men.

The ankh

When the seven planets that were traditionally thought to make up our solar system are plotted outwards from the Sun, Mercury appears as the little courier of the Sun and, beyond him, comes Venus and then the Earth. Venus and Earth, 'the twin planets' as they are sometimes called, are the body and the material world. Venus, goddess of love and beauty, governs all things sensual while Earth, or Mother Nature, is the womb or the home of mortal life. When the cross is set within the circle instead of below it, the symbol for Earth is formed.

A cross in a circle is a wheel. The 'invention' of the wheel is inseparable from the formation and development of humanity. The turning wheel provides the velocity for energy to be channelled and used. It has been the basis of all our material progress, whether through water, wind, clockwork or steam power. The wheel gives us not only the means to progress materially but to develop spiritually. A wheel is a chakra through which energy is drawn in and put out. The four spokes and four chambers provide the conflict of polarity that is necessary for progress.

The cross gives us the polarities of direction and time: it is the basis of the compass and the clock. It points out the four directions and the four corners of Earth, the four elements, the seasons and winds. It gives us choice, or the illusion of it. At the cross-roads we must select a direction but, within the state of four, of division, one never sees the whole picture. Like Oedipus, who unwittingly killed his father at a fork or cross-roads, we think we are in possession of all the facts but our free choice leads us only to reaffirm our destinies.

The cross is the place of suffering, repentance, forgiveness and transformation. The four polarities of Earth arise from the combination of the horizontal and vertical. The horizontal plane, moving from east to west, divides upper from lower and provides a platform that gives breadth and support for all that lives on Earth. It is where the Sun, Moon and planets rise and set. It is where we begin and end. Below the horizon is night, the subconscious and the underworld; above it is day and consciousness. The Hermetic adage of the alchemists, 'As above, so below' was written on the mythological Emerald Tablet, the green platform of Earth and of the heart chakra.

The vertical divides east from west and so creates right and left, or right and wrong. Left comes from Old English and means weak or worthless while in Latin the word for left, 'sinister', implies 'evil'; 'right', on the other hand, is 'right'. Whereas the horizontal gives an undifferentiated embrace to all creatures, the vertical represents the individual. In the spiritual thinking associated with the concept of polarity, the underworld, the unconscious, the night and the dark, the left and the sinister are all related to the feminine. Day, light, consciousness, right, and reason are related to the masculine. Not surprisingly, many people, men as well as women, feel an aversion to this way of thinking when they encounter it and many of the evils of the world can be placed at the doorstep of this body of thought.

But polarity exists whether we like it or not. We can see it wherever we look. The binary system of a circle and a line or a nought and a one is the basis of our computer technology. The philosopher Liebniz is credited with the formation of the binary system but he himself acknowledged the influence of Taoism, the ancient Chinese thinking that encompassed the philosophy of yin and yang.

According to Taoist thought, the circle represents heaven while the square is representative of Earth. The square is the stage, the place where we act out our suffering and redemption. On a square, vision is limited. Human beings throughout time have attempted to get a better view. To do this involves other geometric shapes. The four symbols - the circle, semicircle, triangle and square - are the basis of all geometry and each can be linked to one of the first four numbers, planets and elements. The circle, the ancient symbol of heaven, is equivalent to number one and to the Sun or element of fire. The semicircle relates to the Moon and water while the triangle has an affinity with three, with Mercury and air and the square links to the number four, to Venus and the planet and element of Earth.

The arrogance of our contemporary belief that the 'discovery' that the Earth is round came, like the 'discovery' of the Americas, only a few generations back, is laughable. The Earth has been presented as square throughout time (with or without elephants and other deities to hold up its corners) not because it is 'really' or materially square but because square, level, flat and four-cornered are of its symbolic nature.

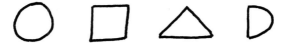

To see the Earth as round requires distance. Because our culture is so materially obsessed, we get that distance through technology - we can now see the Earth as round from photographs taken from satellites. But spiritual devotees of all cultures have always known that it is possible and easy to reach a perspective from which the Earth appears round through the practice of meditation which takes one beyond the polarity of the square and the cross, beyond the mortal body into a place where there is no division, no time or space. The material evidence is still standing of spiritual practices which used geometry to relate the physical, four-cornered plane to the spiritual state of roundness. Homes, temples and even offices in the east are still built so that their cornerstones relate to the positions of the stars in the heavens. Stone circles and ancient temples throughout the world show an alignment of Earth to heaven and the pyramids, it seems, were constructed to align with specific stars.

Looked at from above, the pyramid is like an envelope, its triangles rising to a central point from the the square plane of Earth; the two vertical triangles form a shape like an hour glass while the two horizontal ones are shaped like wings. The hour glass represents time and mortality and the wings suggest transformation, the movement beyond mortal existence and its

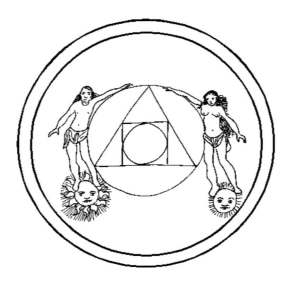

Squaring the circle. Europe. 17th century

limitations. The four triangles together are a geometric representation of the four chambers of the heart.

The heart chakra is not only associated with the heart but with the thymus gland. In a new born baby the thymus is a large gland but it gradually dwindles in size until, at about puberty, it scarcely exists. But, though the gland may have gone, the energy around it remains very strong.

The thymus gland is responsible for building up the immune system. A new-born baby derives its immunity through its mother's milk but, once it is weaned, it has to build up its own immunity to all that may threaten it. The fact that we need to develop immunity to exist on Earth suggests that we are not primarily of the Earth. Immunity comes about through experience and suffering. It is in early childhood when one is first exposed to disease, that immunity is formed and it is also during early childhood that one is especially susceptible to the influence of other people.

The way in which the immune system develops is closely related to the way one learns to think. Unclear feelings of guilt, shame and duty developed early in life make free choice impossible and many chest problems such as asthma and bronchial trouble are found in children who are highly sensitive and who suffer from a feeling of intellectual or emotional oppression from the adults or older children around them.

The white of innocence, symbolised in the dove, the lamb, the lily, nymph and virgin, mixes with the red of experience and suffering when it is incarnated in the flesh. Blood itself is made of white and red corpuscles, the white being those responsible for developing immunity.

Experience is symbolised by the cross of sacrifice, the crown of thorns and the red rose. Through experience we gain compassion and compassion can never be forced. It comes from the heart and is seen in the aura as pink. The heart as the centre of the cross is the place of sacrifice and wisdom. At the heart one has a chance to confess and atone. It is said that the heart is looked into at the Day of Judgement and weighed against a feather, symbol of airy lightness, of freedom from matter and sin.

The condition of being human is, it would seem, venomous and sinful. We are fallen from grace. But were we pushed or did we jump? Why should spirit, living in a state of Paradise, bother to descend to Earth, to a condition of division and struggle? The answer seems to be that through the body, through life on Earth, development or evolution can take place.

Adam and Eve, like many other polarities of masculine and feminine, represent spirit and matter. Matter, then, is born from the rib of spirit and the ribs are the ladder of evolution. Evolution can only take place through experience and to gain experience, one must be made of flesh and blood, one must partake of the symbol of the cross, of mortality and suffering, and descend to incarnate into the flesh, Venus (or Aphrodite), and to life on the Earth, Gaia.

After the fall, the task of mankind and of the whole of nature is to attain again, through the wisdom that comes from experience, the state of grace. In reverse, the first four letters of 'evolve' spell 'love', and the word 'evil' in reverse is 'live'. Merely to live is to sin, to experience without learning or growth. To evolve, one has to transcend the individual ego and love.

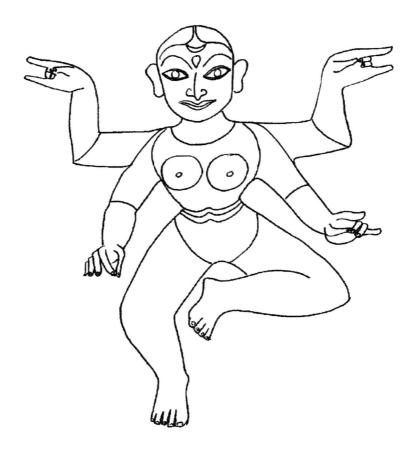

The goddess, Jagadamba, the Mother of the World. Bengal. 18th century.

An exercise

Sit with your spine straight. Bring your awareness to the G-spot or perineum point. (See the exercise at the end of chapter 2: The Pituitary, page 37.)

Come up the inside of the body to the heart chakra in the centre of the chest.

Find the heart chakra as a wheel on the spine and try to sense its energy coming forward out of the body.

Return to the G-spot or perineum point. Rest there.

Go back up to the heart chakra and rest there.

Continue the movement up and down, resting at each position.

Finish after ten or fifteen minutes at the heart chakra.

Five
The Sun

The Solar Plexus

*'In the circle
of Being, only
you are.'*

Awhaduddin Kermani

According to myth, we have fallen from grace. Tempted by the snake to the pleasures of the flesh, we find ourselves, beautiful, free spirits that we really are, trapped in mortal bodies on the dull flat plain of Earth. Some religions even go so far as to say that all matter - everything on Earth and the Earth

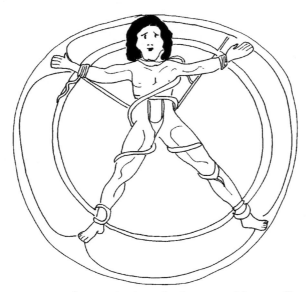

Ixion tied to a spinning wheel as a punishment. Greece

itself - is the product of the devil. It is the terrain of the evil Eve and the venomous Venus.

As long as we are condemned to the wheel of life, we turn on the cross of suffering. And yet it is the cross that brings redemption and the opportunity to make our weary way back to our celestial home, bedraggled and exhausted but humbled, loving and wise. The cross is, of course, the symbol of sacrifice and we can only wend our way back to Paradise through the sacrifice of our mortal bodies and of our attachment to the Earth and life in material form. Most current religions describe Earth as female and heaven as male. All of us, men and women alike, are of the spirit but incarnated in flesh. We spend our lives on the level of the female: we are made of matter or Mater and derive our sustenance from Mother Nature but only when we truly understand that the material world is illusory, do we regain our spiritual home.

Patriarchal religions declare that the spiritual life cannot be attained by women. Buddhists believe that Nirvana or Paradise can only be reached through incarnation in a male body, not so long ago, male Christians took it upon themselves to determine whether or not women had souls (concluding, by a small margin that they do but that animals don't), and numerous religions deem women unfit to be priests since their bodies are sexual and therefore sinful.

There have been plenty of women throughout history ready to accept that they are evil and must be punished, humiliated and restrained. The little girl who, aged four or five, has every bone in her feet broken and bound to ensure they can never heal learns it is bad to want to walk or run and she is bad to have the urge to do so. The girl who has her sexual organs ritually mutilated learns it is bad to have sexual feelings or preferences. The girl who sees her mother beaten and nobody interfering learns that women deserve to be punished. And only a few generations back, in our own society, those girls who watched their mothers, aunts and grandmothers strapped to the ducking stool and submerged in filthy water, a punishment that frequently resulted in drowning, learned that an independent or outspoken woman was not to be tolerated.

Girls have learned early on that females have to be punished and restricted. Since those who carry out the punishments and impose the fetters are fathers, mothers, men of religion, doctors, lawyers, grandmothers and other

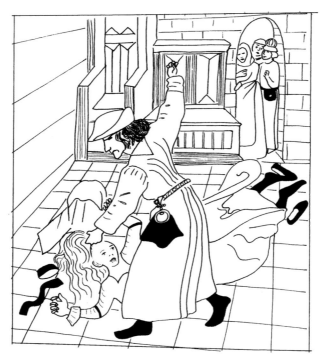

Wife beating. Europe. Sixteenth century.

elders of the community, there is no doubt in the girls' minds that punishment and restraint are necessary and deserved. Masochism is imbibed with mother's milk - indeed, many girls never even make it to imbibe mother's milk, the widespread infanticide of baby girls having been superseded by the more efficient method of aborting foetuses for the crime of being female. It is hardly surprising that masochism seems to belong to the female nature and that women, even when offered the chance to escape from abuse, frequently do not accept it.

But, somehow or other, women do manage to go on expressing themselves in patriarchal cultures. Though little survives in print or on canvas, myths go on forever.

Fairy stories tell of change and transformation. The frog or beast turns into a prince and the serving girl becomes a queen. These are stories about

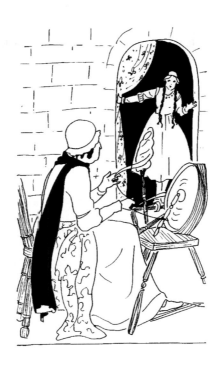

Spinster. Europe. Twentieth century.

growing up; about attaining the state of grace - the ugly duckling becomes a pure white swan; and about reaching heaven, the place where opposites are joined in union as symbolised in the royal wedding. Such stories describe the alchemical process. When transformation takes place in nature, the butterfly or nymph emerges from the chrysalis. It is in the chrysalis that change takes place and 'chrysalis' itself means 'gold' or 'of the Sun'. From it comes chrysanthemum, 'the golden flower' whose unfolding conforms to the 'golden spiral', and allied to it are the shining ones: Christ and Krishna.

The chrysalis is a spun container of gossamer thread that looks like a spindle and seems to hold light. In nature, it is the female that spins the chrysalis and in human life, too, it is traditionally women who spin. In fairy stories the spinners (or spinsters as they used to be known) are the old or childless women. Though they are not at the centre of action, they have a grave responsibility for the destinies of the community. When the pubescent girl encounters the old woman and attempts to spin she pricks her finger, blood is released and she falls down as if dead only to be woken by sexual contact and union with the prince.

The death of the Sleeping Beauty echoes the death of Christ. Both are much-loved children heralded at birth as special. They are encircled by a group of twelve, one of whom, the betrayer, causes blood to be spilled and the hero or heroine appears to be lost. But they rise again, awakening with them an entourage of followers. The palace, the society, the whole of humanity is saved by the death and rebirth of the heroine or hero.

The ability to spin is the ability to bring about change and to create something of value. The young woman locked in a room and commanded to spin straw into gold is required to prove herself as an alchemist and to show herself worthy to be the king's wife and capable of creating the cocoon in which to gestate a child. Being female involves bodily change. The young princess emerges from her own pupahood, her chrysalis form, to become a nymph and, in the process, discharges blood, thereby proving her sexuality and fertility as well as her mortality. The king's young bride has to create the conditions for pregnancy; she has to develop from nymph to queen.

Traditionally, puberty when menstruation begins and the inner labia, the nympha, develop and open, was the time that the nymph was caught in the net of wife and motherhood. When the entrance to the womb opened at puberty, the young girl would emerge from the thalamus where she had lived protected by the mothers into the nymphon or marriage chamber where, under the supervision of the god, Hymen, she would be 'deflowered'.

'Nymphon' means not only 'marriage chamber' but also 'sea-spider'. So, the nymph or pia mater would, on her marriage in the nymphon, be transformed into the spinner of the chrysalis, the weaver of destinies, the fertile mother, the arachnoid mater. Like the nymphon, the nymph was, and still is, adorned with net or lace, reflecting the state of illusion, the condition of Maya, the great goddess who contains all potential. The virgin nymph behind the veil is in the state of perfection but when the veil is lifted by her husband, symbolising the breaking of the hymen, she emerges into what we know as the real world but what is, in fact, the state of illusion.

The nymph, on marriage, promises fidelity and obedience but if, like Venus, she breaks her wedding vows, she may find herself netted again. To be of the flesh and of the world is to be subject to deception and illusion and nowhere is deception more practised than in the arena of sex. Venus herself was not above sexual deception and, when found out, suffered a particularly nasty and embarrassing experience trapped in a net fashioned by her husband, Hephaestus.

Hephaestus was as ugly as sin but was elevated to Mount Olympus and to marriage with the beautiful Aphrodite or Venus on account of his great skill as a smith. He made countless invaluable and useful objects for the gods and, for his own purposes made a net so fine it was invisible in which he trapped Venus and her lover Mars and then displayed them naked for all the gods to see.

As smith, Hephaestus, (or Vulcan in his Roman form) plays with fire but, unlike so many would-be heroes, he has learned to control the fire and make it work for him. He has created culture and art out of raw energy.

The fire of the Sun is our basic creative material and handling it correctly enables us to purify ourselves of our base emotional greed to become accepted by the gods themselves. Fire has to be treated with respect and the attempt to make gold or to reach the Sun can be dangerous. Gold is the reward of the humble. You reach it through simplicity and trust as Jack got the golden egg, harp and coins by planting a humble bean. You have to earn your gold. If you take it when it is not due to you, you will suffer. King Midas, who wished that everything he touched might turn to gold, discovered, when even his dinner and his daughter turned to gold, that it was a cold, unfeeling substance.

The journey to the Sun is the voyage through the ego to the self, a progression that requires moderation, discipline and caution. The ego can cause destruction not only of the individual but of the universe. There are plenty of warnings in myth. Many of the stories of tampering with solar energies involve fathers and sons; the son may interfere with his father's energy before he has learned the lessons of handling his own or the father may be overly ambitious for his son, as was Dedalus for Icarus.

Dedalus made wings of wax for both himself and his son, Icarus, but the youthful and over-enthusiastic Icarus flew too near the Sun and, of course, his wings melted. Wax is not the best material for solar flying; it is the substance of effigies. Those who make their wings of wax suffer from delusions of grandeur.

Pride came before a fall, too, when Phaeton took his father's, Apollo's, horses and drove the Sun wildly through the sky, setting fire to the Earth and endangering the universe, causing the necessity for his own destruction. In myth, the Sun is the father and to usurp the father's power without having earned it is to ask for trouble. Prometheus stole fire from his father and was condemned to lie on a rock under the hot Sun for evermore with a black bird pecking his liver, life itself, all day. Ego can be a driving creative force or one that is consuming and destructive in its hunger for power but we cannot ignore it. The Buddha gave it all the attention he could, saying that, only by developing the ego could one get free of its domination. Solar energy, or fire, is a pulsation, consistent and reliable but, when its rhythm suffers interference, it is liable to flare out of control. The task of the hero or heroine is to become king or queen by marrying the princess or prince or by achieving solar - or spiritual status - through their own courage, ingenuity and persistence.

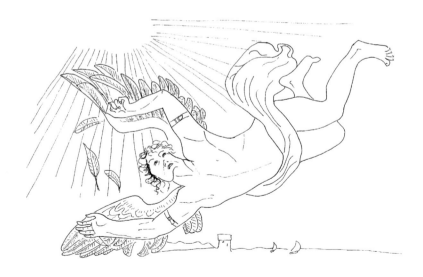

Icarus

To be king or queen is to be one's own authority, to be the centre of one's world, to be the Sun. This is a position fraught with the dangers of arrogance, pride and over-ambition, all of which were characteristics of the self-styled Roi Soleil, the Sun King, Louis X1V, whose unlimited personal greed caused starvation, decadence and appalling suffering.

The French for sun, 'soleil', comes from the Latin, 'sol' which gives rise to words that suggest oneness and even aloneness - solo, solitary, solitude and isolation. Within the body, the solar plexus is the centre; 'solar' means sun and 'plexus' means a meeting of nerves. The Sun, radiating light and heat at the centre of our planetary system, is found in replica in the centre of the body radiating energy through the nerves. The state of solitude is very different from that of loneliness. Solitude brings peace and a sense of belonging. It is the condition of love that goes beyond emotional wants to acceptance of things as they are.

A healthy solar plexus is a golden yellow and radiates warmth. It is as steady as the Sun, unaffected by the emotions of others but, frequently, the solar plexus can be experienced as charred, burned out and blackened as a consequence of fear. Fear often makes us withdraw and the solar plexus may feel more like a black hole than a radiating source of energy.

Related to the solar plexus is the pancreas which secretes digestive juices and is responsible for breaking down food and changing it into energy. The effect of its actions is to increase the blood sugar, thereby creating sweetness. Digestion is affected by anxiety and fear, sweetness can turn to acidity and bitterness, and indigestion can be experienced as a burning that is out of control. Sweetness is found in sugar and in honey, both terms of endearment and love. Sweetbreads are delicacies made from the pancreas or thymus glands of animals, the glands associated with the heart and solar plexus chakras, centres of joy and love.

Like heat, energy rises and the ancient transmutation practices performed by monks involve moving energy up the spine to the level of the solar plexus where, through the element of fire, it changes and, as it continues its upward movement, arriving at the heart level, it is transformed through the element of air, providing freedom from Earthly bonds.

These eastern practices have similarities in the practice of alchemy, the attempt to change base metal into gold. Base metal or matter is the Earth;

gold is the Sun. The Earth is identified with the square, the cross and the number four while the Sun is identified with the five-pointed star, with centrality, steadiness, power and regulation.

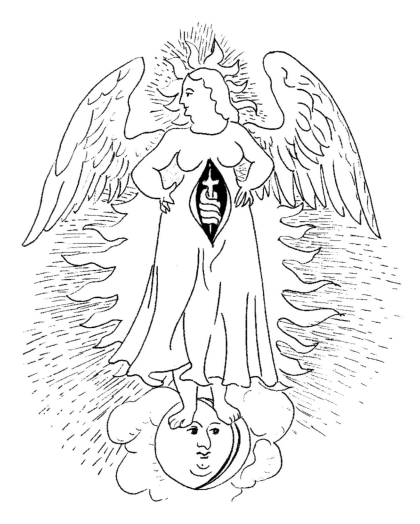

Through the transmutation of energy at the solar plexus the state of divinity is reached. Europe. 16th century.

Tables and chairs are four legged but have no heads. If they did they would no longer be the useful supports that they are. They would have minds of their own and would never be there when you wanted them. Creatures that walk on four legs are attached to Earth and they do not have the possibility of transcendence. They cannot create change; they may resist capture and taming but they cannot plan a revolution and must live by the existing order. But the number five offers the opportunity for change and elevation.

The fifth limb, the head, provides the exercise of mind over matter, the possibility of free-will. And man, standing as he does on his two dainty feet, rising upwards, bold and brave, to the Sun, is the image of the five-pointed star. Through the exercise of his mind, he can tame nature and subdue it, he can create culture and civilisation, he can elevate himself to the stature of the gods.

The solar plexus is the position of change and exchange and five is the number of balance, harmony and culture. The first four numbers added together make ten; one, two, three and four make a unit complete in itself. But number five is a star, an explosion of light, a new beginning. Five gathers the four corners to a central point. It is the still centre of the four winds and the four directions. It spins the four elements into ether, the background of the universe. It is said that for the first three minutes of the universe there was no number five. The four nuclei that make the atom found stability but then the fifth came along and caused a massive explosion. Through the ensuing chaos a new order came about. What was created from the Big Bang was the universe, a system of an infinite number of stars, constantly moving, constantly changing. Each star comes from the original void, the place of unity beyond division. If, therefore, we wish to return to the source of all things, we have to go via the stars.

Five - two plus three - is the fundamental proportion of what is considered to be the perfect form achievable by man. 'Sol' is the fifth note of the musical scale and five produces the Golden Section, Triangle, Spiral, Measurement, Mean and so on. These harmonious structures were not only the foundations of classical art and design but also constituted the basis of Egyptian civilisation.

The Sun, related both to the head and the pineal chakra (see chapter one) and to the solar plexus and the central area of the human being, is the place of government, understanding and balance. From it comes regulation and control. It is an exchange, setting the standard value. While kings and other representatives of nations are busy putting their own heads on their currencies and calling their coins 'sovereigns' or 'crowns', they and their nations wealth are susceptible to fluctuations of value. But gold remains unaffected by the stock markets, beyond the vagaries of ego and time.

'Helios', the word for 'Sun' in Latin and Greek, means 'the centre of a spiral' (proving that the ancients knew full well that the Sun was the centre of a planetary system) and related to it are 'helix' which means not only a coil but the common snail and the rim of the ear; and 'heliconia', a family of butterflies that shares its name with the Greek Muses who come from Mount Helicon and are the constant companions of Apollo. The ancients believed that the Sun not only put out energy but drew back into itself the

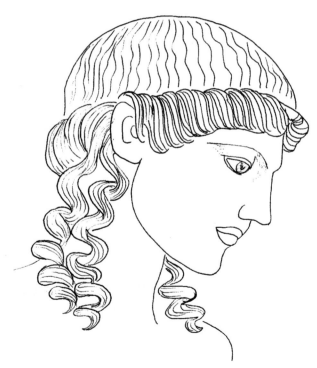

Apollo Chrysocomes, 'of the golden locks'. Greek

pollution and waste that life produced. Certainly, if you look at a setting Sun on a clear still evening, you see its dimming rays appear to be moving in towards itself. The only safe way to dispose of nuclear waste is to send it back to the Sun. Just as the Sun devours arrogance and pride, so it will absorb their products.

A partner exercise

Sit opposite your partner. Both partners are to work at the same time. Close your eyes and make contact with your solar plexus chakra, a wheel of energy on the front of the spine.

From there, bring the energy out towards your partner's solar plexus chakra.

Rest there and try to sense it.

Then bring the energy from your partner's solar plexus into the space between you.

Both partners can now try to sense what is happening between them.

If you get confused about what is yours and what is your partner's, return to your own solar plexus chakra and repeat the exercise.

Finish after ten or fifteen minutes by returning to your own solar plexus chakra.

Share with your partner your experience.

Six
Mars   The Hara

> *'Vast is Heaven's net*
> *sparse-meshed it is, and yet*
> *nothing can slip through it.'*
>
> Lao Tsu

The most famous of the artefacts Hephaestus created was his net, so strong it could trap immortals but so fine it could not be seen. Because it was never seen, there is no record of what it looked like. But for a net to be strong, it lends itself to be made of either three or six sides and the six-sided mesh is the fabric of the cellular structure that can be identified with Mars, the humiliated lover of Venus, trapped in his rival's net.

In many European languages the words for six and sex overlap. Six is the number of fertility and 'the number of the beast' in popular myth is 666. The beast and the devil are one and the same, they are tempters of the flesh, akin to Eve and Venus to whom Mars was irresistibly attracted. (The antidote to temptation, it should never be forgotten, is to call 999, the number of the police and the head, the male force of reason and logic.)

A six-sided shape, or hexagon, makes the form of a cell.

Cells joined together can be seen in a honeycomb which is composed of a pattern of hexagons forming a strong and flexible structure which can be

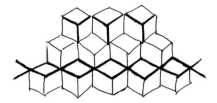

added to indefinitely. A honeycomb has two identical walls which reinforce each other, their cells overlapping so that, alternating with each X shape made by two adjoining hexagons, is a Y shape that is made by the backing wall. In the pattern made by the cell walls lie the forms of the X and Y chromosomes, the basic structure of life, the X acting as the link between the cells which contain the Y.

The bee has been worshipped as the source of all good things. The queen bee is, perhaps, the most fertile of all creatures and the whole community works to support her. The cells of the honeycomb are actually chambers in which the eggs are nourished by the nurse bees. The bee appears to have no ego. Everything it does is for the sake of the community. It responds to higher vibrations than we are aware of, its colour range beginning with our blues and violets. It is tempting to suggest that it is, therefore, a more spiritual creature and it has certainly been treated as such in many societies. Blues and violets are associated with the head. Blue belongs to the throat or thyroid chakra, indigo to the pineal or third eye, and purple to the crown. They are colours of healing, penetration and devotion. Any healer who is capable of working at the deep level necessary for helping overcome serious illnesses like cancer and arthritis will have violet as a prominent colour in the aura. Anyone who has the true calling of priest, whether or not they are officially recognised, will show the colour purple.

The bee penetrates the flower with its proboscis but it does not enter the receptacle, the sacred thalamus or inner chamber. It goes no further, metaphorically, than the nymphon or bridal chamber, fertilising the flower though the transfer of pollen which it collects from the stamen of a plant. The word stamen refers not only to the male part of the plant but to the thread spun by the Fates at the time of a person's birth. The stamen is the warp of the weaving, the upright strand, the principle of individuation while the bee creates the blend, the woof to the warp, through the mingling of

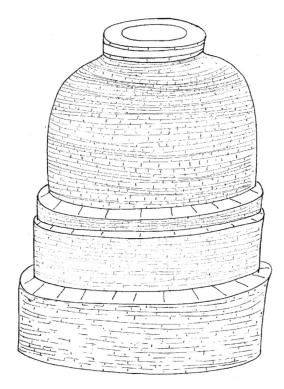

Beehive-shaped temple. Ecuador.

pollen and the creation of honey. Honey is the food of love, it is the sexual juices and, intriguingly, the word 'semen' comes from the word for six. A 'semester', which is now a university or college term, originally meant a period of six months.

Semen is the fluid that carries the seed and 'to seminate' means to sow. The sower of seeds is Mars. God's command to 'be fruitful and multiply', given on the sixth day, the day on which he created 'the beast of the Earth and everything that creepeth upon the Earth', including man, is put into practice by Mars who is primarily god of agriculture.

According to the Bible, the first race and, therefore, the 'seminal' one, is that descended from David: the Semites. The House of David is represented by the six-pointed star, formed by two equilateral triangles, one pointing up, the other down.

The Star of David

It is known as a hexagram, the word which also describes the six lines of the oracle of the I Ching, the ancient Chinese 'Book of Changes'. The up-pointing triangle represents the male force while the down-pointing one is female. The two together create in their centre the cell-shaped hexagon, fertility itself.

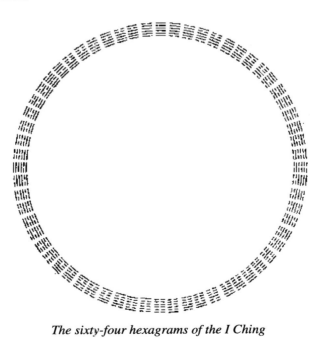

The sixty-four hexagrams of the I Ching

The six lines of the hexagrams of the I Ching show all the potential between Earth and Heaven and, therefore, all relationships between human beings.

The orbit of Mars lies the other side of the Earth from Venus so it is through or on Earth, the planet of love, sometimes identified with the Sun, that the loving couple interact. The creatures of Earth are, in a sense, the children of Venus and Mars and, if Venus can be seen as Eve, then Mars can be associated with Adam. Mars is the scatterer of seeds, the sower of wild oats. But he is not just a Don Juan. He is concerned to care for his progeny. From the word 'semen' comes 'seminary' which is a plot of land where seeds are planted and nursed and a seminary is also a place where monks and nuns devote themselves to cultivating the seeds of ideas.

Mars is not only god of agriculture but of war and God's command is not only to 'replenish the Earth' but to 'subdue it'. Sexuality and conquest, even in God's mind, are related. The practice of agriculture has brought about the manufacture of ever more sophisticated machinery, much of which appears to be making war, not love, to the Earth. Wars, traditionally, are fought between men for possession of women and land. Mars husbands both woman and the Earth but the impulse of Mars, when uncontrolled, can become an anarchy of rape. The Martian impulse to conquer and to make one's mark can be seen not only in agriculture but in exploration. Climbers, for instance, still talk about 'assaulting' a rock face or 'conquering' Everest. And the achievement of the individual male in mastering a piece of nature or space is still attributed to his nation as if the whole tribe had gone to war in his person.

The identification of Mars with conquest and military performance led to the assumption that the planet Mars itself was technologically advanced. Until comparatively recently astronomers 'saw' straight lines on Mars which, some concluded, were canals and therefore provided evidence that Mars was inhabited. Today this seems just another fantasy masquerading as science but there was, in fact, good reason to assume that Mars had undergone an industrial revolution.

Mars's drive to fertilise, propagate and conquer leads to the desire to improve on the efficiency of nature. As god of agriculture, Mars is, by extension, ruler of the market place, or 'mart', to which he has given his name. At his worst, he is the farmer who will stop at nothing to make his land more profitable, confusing husbandry with warfare. Mars is the god of discipline, order and control and has given his name, too, to all things martial.

As god of war, Mars requires the individual to subjugate himself to the state. The loyal subject is asked to suppress his will for the benefit of the community. The able-bodied male, in times of war, is expected to fit into his role without questioning the purpose. To fight for his country is a sign of his manhood and a male proves himself through his potency, his semen. The connections between warfare and masculine potency are well documented: bullets scattered from guns, bombs ejected from planes to fall into the Earth below, the taunts sung by soldiers to undermine the enemy, such as the World War II ditty, 'Hitler's only got one ball; Goering's got two but very small'.

The energy of Mars can, when it is based on insecurity, be weak, domineering, taunting, irritable, frustrated, angry and out of control. But when it is based on security, it can be motivated, controlled, assertive, confident, directed, purposeful. In other words, it is the will.

Through the will, one exercises free choice. One determines, or has the illusion of determining, one's fate. The will is the male sexual organ and represents power and potency. There is no arguing with the will: 'Thy will be done'. A will gives instructions to be implemented after one's death. It determines how the harvest of one's life will be disseminated, how one's seeds will continue to bear fruit and to whom one's profits will be awarded.

When the will is strong it is said to be made of iron and it is not surprising that iron is the metal that is associated with Mars. You can still see the symbol for Mars in some ironmongers, just as you can see the intertwining snakes of Mercury's caduceus in some chemist shops. The Egyptians believed that comets hitting the Earth brought with them iron which was the semen of the gods to fertilise the Earth. Perhaps the net that trapped Mars and Venus for all to see was formed of hexagonals and forged of iron by the smith of the gods.

The energy of the will is derived from the hara chakra, situated just below the navel. 'Hara' is a Sanskrit word meaning 'soul'. Unlike the other chakras, the hara does not receive energy directly from the spleen chakra but is dependent on the root chakra below it. (See Chapter 8). The colour related to the hara is orange, a mixture of the red which belongs to the root

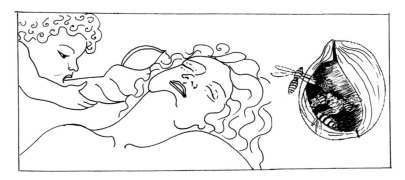

The famous Botticelli painting of Mars and Venus shows, next to the sexually exhausted Mars, a hive of wasps, of the genus hymenoptera.

chakra and of the yellow of the solar plexus. Its element is water and water can be the calmest thing in the world or the most disturbed.

In dreams, water reflects the emotional state: murky water, for instance, shows unclear emotions, a deep pool shows profundity of feeling, a stormy sea indicates troubled thoughts, and so on. A person going through an emotional release may experience a discharge of water. They may, for example, sweat at night, have a wet dream or even wet the bed. Relaxation of the body will always produce a release of water and it is common in meditation, as in sleep, to find an excess of saliva produced in the mouth. Water is the strongest thing in the world and the most humble. It is a female element and its tendency is downwards.

> *'Why is the sea king of a hundred streams?*
> *Because it lies below them.*
> *Therefore it is king of a hundred streams.'*

> Lao Tsu

The glands associated with the hara are the adrenals which are situated on the kidneys and work to collect and expel water from the body. The adrenals release adrenalin, the flight or fight hormone. When a person is stimulated, say by shock or sexual excitement, a rush of the hormone gives the body the opportunity to react. It is this hormone that is responsible for both the impulse to attack and to make love. It is easy to see how the two can become confused and easy to understand how soldiers called upon to destroy and kill, build up the urge to rape as well, to 'replenish the Earth and subdue it'.

Since the energy of the hara is dependent on that of the root, the glands associated with both chakras are also intimately connected. The glands identified with the root chakra are the ovaries and testes while the highly emotional area of the hara is related to the expression of sexuality, to the menstrual cycle and to the cycle of the formation and release of semen.

The hara area of the body is the motor area. Energy from the hara is drawn on in performing everyday tasks such as driving a car or washing up. Such simple tasks can become a focus for aggression and anger: the car can turn into a weapon; who does or doesn't do the washing up can become an issue that destroys relationships. The anger and frustration registered at the hara chakra may, in fact, stem from feelings of impotence which have their origin in the sexual organs and the root chakra. Such anger may at times find its release in sexuality and the sexual act can become an arena for the release of frustration rather than the expression of love.

Like all the endocrine glands, the adrenals are subject to the pituitary. While the impulse from the adrenals relates to instinct and, in a sense, to the animal part of ourselves, the pituitary, located in the centre of the brain, is influenced by thought. Conflict between the emotions and patterns of thinking may take its toll on the body and contribute to a sense of being out of control. But when thought is at one with instinctual behaviour, both body and mind are fertile and at peace.

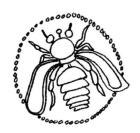

An exercise

Sit with the spine straight and close your eyes.

Bring your awareness to the hara chakra on the front of the spine.
(The hara is situated four fingers breadth below the navel.) Allow
yourself to be drawn into the chakra.

When you have made a good contact, feel the energy coming
forwards beyond the body.

Then move out of the front of the body up to the pineal chakra on the
forehead. Allow yourself to be drawn in.

After a minute or two come back out of the forehead to the hara
chakra. Allow yourself to be drawn in.

Repeat this movement for a ten or fifteen minute period, finishing at
the hara.

It can also be beneficial to contact the hara when taking a bath or
swimming and to feel the energy come forwards and expand
outwards in ripples.

Seven
Jupiter   The Crown

> *'There is a tide in the affairs of men which*
> *taken at the flood, leads on to fortune...*
> *we must take the current when it serves,*
> *or lose our ventures'.*
>
> William Shakespeare

There are some insects that only fly once. They break out of the chrysalis, spread their wings and fly to the spot where they will mate, lay their eggs and die. And so it is with some human nymphs. Like Cinderella, they emerge from the basement, put on their glad rags, go to the ball, fall for the prince and live happily ever after confined within the palace walls.

The girl pricks her finger on a spindle (instrument for making cocoons), sheds blood and breaks out of her pupa, or cocoon, to become a nymph. The nymph is seduced by the king and, by spinning straw into gold and so making a new chrysalis or pupa, she becomes queen and gestates a child.

The queen of the insects forsakes freedom for fertility and its demands of stillness, darkness and centrality. Her abode is the women's room, the dark heart of the society, the secluded receptive place where eggs are fertilised and hatched. For the first seven days of her life the Queen Bee is known as the Virgin Queen and is free to fly but, on the seventh day she mates and never flies again. She creates the community and is serviced by it, delivering her offspring into hexagonal cells in the nursery where they are nurtured by the nurse bees. The hierarchy of the bee-hive is natural and essential.

The virgin or nymph was traditionally married in the nymphon but now that the female spiritual tradition has been so thoroughly eradicated that we cannot even remember it, the bride goes to the male church (or its civic counterpart) to be married. She is led up the aisle by her father and handed to the groom who waits symbolically in his place, the heart of the masculine church. Beyond the altar is the head of the church into which only the priests are allowed. Just as ancient temples were laid out to reflect the sacred human body so the Christian church is designed with a head, body and, sometimes, a chapel to each side of the 'heart' representing the arms and so making the form of the cross. The head is the place from which instruction comes to be passed on to the body, the congregation. Only the priests have access to the will or mind of God; beyond the altar is closed shop.

But time was when marriage took place on female territory. The bride was not given away or sold or bartered from father to husband but remained in the place where she had always belonged, with the mothers in the women's quarters. The worship that took place in the nymphon was not the worship of the head, or of the word as it is in the masculine church, but worship of the womb, the home, the intuition, of nature and fertility.

The meeting of male and female in the nymphon brought about the intermingling of complementary energies. The male, belonging to the outside world, and the female, belonging to the inner, met in the sacred nymphon that led to the inner sanctum, in the symbolic vagina that provides the only entrance to the sanctum of the womb in the form of the miniscule aperture known as the cervix, the same word that describes the bones in the neck linking head and body. That the correspondance between the womb and the centre of the head was acknowledged in the past is shown in the Latin word for thalamus, 'gynaecium'. Gynaecium has the same meanings as thalamus: the sacred chamber, the receptacle of the flower, the centre of the head, the women's rooms and it also means the womb.

The union of male and female, one and two, Narcissus and Echo, brings the possiblity of procreation and allows the number three to come into being. The female transformation that takes place at puberty involves the opening of the inner labia or nympha to allow for the sexual act. In birth the baby's head descends the birth canal and pushes open the inner labia to meet the outer. When it reaches its fullness it is said to 'crown'.

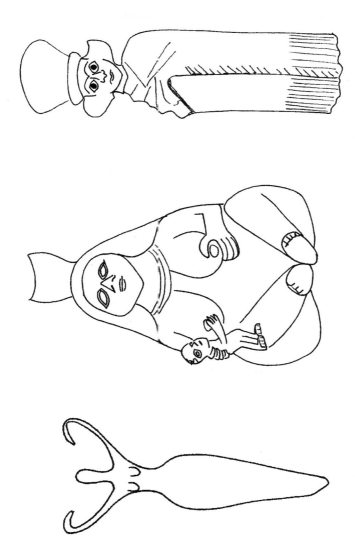

Dura Mater
Old goddess or crone

Arachnoid Mater
Fertile goddess

Pia Mater
Young and slender goddess

87

The crowning (which occurs at ten centimetres or five fingers' dilation) refers to both mother and baby. The baby's head is crowned by the birth canal and the mother is crowned in that she has become queen. (Cats become queens as soon as they fall pregnant). Through pregnancy and birth, she has graduated from nymph or virgin to crone, a word that once, far from having the negative connotations it has today, meant 'corona' or 'crown'.

Human life cycles, like those of insects, have several stages of transformation. The process of transformation is related to the number seven. Seven is the turning point when one stage is finished and the next is about to begin.

'All movements are accomplished in six stages', says the I Ching, 'and the seventh brings return. Thus the winter solstice, with which the decline of the year begins, comes in the seventh month after the summer solstice; so too sunrise comes in the seventh double hour after sunset. Therefore seven is the number of the young light, and it arises when six, the number of the great darkness, is increased by one. In this way the state of rest gives place to movement.' (No 24. Fu. Return.)

It is said that every seven years we start anew since, in that time, all the cells in the body are replaced. Not surprising, then, that we experience a 'seven-year itch'. Seven is the age when milk teeth fall out and the adult teeth come through. In many cultures, boys are taken from their mothers at seven. Fourteen, the age of puberty, is the age of initiation when the young person is taken into the religious culture through rituals such as Bar Mitzvah or confirmation. At twenty-one, we are given the key of the door. The number seven appears time and again in mystical traditions. In the Kabbalah, the Hebrew tradition, for instance, the Tree of Life has seven branches each with seven leaves.

The common factor in all the symbolism surrounding the number seven is the division of attainment into stages. Seven is a ladder ascended by each being. It is, therefore, a number of hierarchy while also a number that unites all creatures in common experience. The number seven suggests that all beings have a purpose to fulfil in their own time but not all have reached the same level of attainment. As a ladder, seven is also a scale. The musical scale has seven notes (the eighth being the repetition of the first on a higher vibration) and the rainbow has seven colours. Each of the seven chakras has seven tones to its colour, the central one being the essence of the chakra.

Seven vibrating together make one whole. Seven is the number of richness and strength.

Seven are the seven stars in the sky. The seven stars are not only the seven planets of traditional astrology but are the stars that compose the Great Bear known also as the Plough or Dipper, his smaller brother the Little Bear, Orion whom the Egyptians knew as Osiris, with his four extremities and three-starred belt, and the Seven Sisters or Pleiades. Both the Pleiades and Orion mark areas in the cosmos where stars are born. The birth of a star is not what one might expect, a long drawn-out, difficult process. Stars are spewn out prolifically and continuously.

Seven connects heaven and Earth: it links the three of the triangle with the four of the square and so gives the basic form of the pyramid which is composed of four triangles set on a square base. One of the purposes of the pyramids, it has been suggested, was to aid the spirit of the god to come to Earth to be incarnated in the body of the king and, on the king's death, to enable the spirit to return to its home in the skies.

Seven, then, is the number of manifestation. Through it, spirit becomes lodged in matter and thoughts become deeds. It is a mystical or magical number, the number of psychic ability. I once met a seventh daughter of a seventh daughter who gave me a four-leafed clover, painted silver, from a collection she had made simply by knowing when she would find one in the grass at her feet. Such superficial words as 'luck', 'coincidence' and

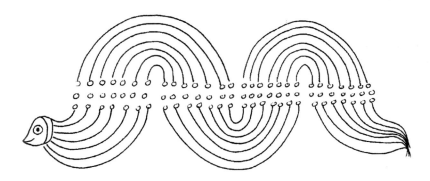

The sevenfold universe. India. 19th century.

'chance' have a deeper meaning and seven is not merely a lucky number. It has profound spiritual significance.

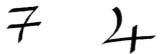

Back-to-front and upside-down, seven makes the symbol for Jupiter, king of the gods, the force behind the laws of nature. Natural laws say that all things are related; one thing is due to another, each effect has a cause, the harvest results from the sowing of seeds. And, similarly, all material forms are the results of thoughts, they are 'the word made flesh'. Jupiter, as king, has the ultimate authority. His word goes. His thoughts and seeds are inseparable, they spill out everywhere sprouting new growth and myriad forms.

Like Mars, Jupiter is concerned with sex, obsessed by it, in fact. His third wife, Juno, is, like her husband, a deity of light and a powerful figure in her own right, but is often portrayed as little more than a frustrated nagging wife, bitterly complaining while her husband is out seducing everyone - nymphs, mortal women, goddesses, as well as attractive males. Though goddess of marriage and childbirth, Juno, belonging to the Roman pantheon, is subject to patriarchal law and is powerless to withstand her husband's adultery, wife-beating and child-abuse (he throws her child, Hephaestus, from the mountain of Olympus). The marriage of Jupiter and Juno is, not surprisingly for the god of the thunderbolt, tempestuous but storms as well as sunshine are needed for productivity,

Since he is king of the gods, Jupiter achieves his aim. Not all the females he desires are willing and eager to accept him but that does not bother him; he simply turns them into cows, rivers or trees and himself into the wind or another of his myriad disguises and has his way with them.

He can bend and adapt the laws of nature because he has had a hand in making them. He is a master magician, overseeing the implementation of thought into practice on the plane of matter. In our limited way, we frequently see only matter, not energy, only the effects, not the causes. We see the events of our lives as accident, chance, coincidence, misadventure, or luck and take no responsibility for our part in the process. But, to those who choose to be aware, what appears to be bad luck may carry a warning

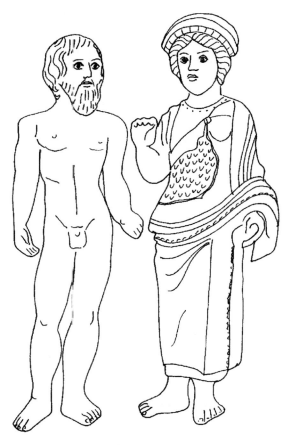

Jupiter and Juno. Etruscan.

or be a result of some previous cause while people who appear to be just lucky types may actually achieve their rewards through intense psychic concentration, through a conscious relationship with the king of the gods.

Such a relationship can be developed through faith, meditation, prayer and ritual, taking us towards an awareness of our own path through life. Just as the Babes in the Wood followed their pebbles home so we can train ourselves to see the signs. Ladders, magpies and ambulances hold general superstitious connotations but true signs are more intimate and personal, referring to our own specific journey, our individual fate. They, like the rainbow, are a communication or link between spirit life and humanity, only appearing when the time and conditions are right so, frequently, taking the form of 'coincidence'. They suggest that there are forces beyond ourselves guiding our lives, encouraging us to find our purpose.

They are like a light in darkness and the task that Jupiter sets us is not only to recognise and follow the signs but to wait in the dark in trust and faith. Despair, doubt and impatience are our downfall but Jupiter requires us to transcend the limitations of our conventional expectations and consequent disappointments, to make fallow times productive, to take courage both in the process of waiting and then in seizing the opportunity offered. Jupiter constantly prompts us to grow beyond ourselves. Recognising and accepting the signs, portents and omens is like embedding the stepping stones or pebbles in the earth.

The key to purposeful action is non-action. Non-action is not passivity but a state of alertness and awareness that comes from the openness brought about by inner calm. We have all come from nothingess, the void is our centre, and yet we find it almost impossible to do and think nothing. We cling to our busy thoughts and activity as if to very life and identity. Finding the faith to wait in incomprehension and nothingness is a challenge met by few. With the Jovian spirit of adventure, however, the fear itself can become a source of amusement. Jupiter is lord of the gamble, overseeing the fluctuations of fortune. Through awareness of his power we can judge when to place our bets and when to withdraw.

We can be aided in understanding the source of the gamble through divination. Drawing the cards, throwing the coins, consulting the tea leaves or the cracked tortoiseshell: these are gambles in themselves, their seeming randomness forming some unseen cosmic pattern. To consult them is to enter into communication with the energies that influence and even create physical life and events on Earth.

Consulting the oracle is a kind of madness necessitating the abandonment of the rational mind. To the true gambling spirit it is compelling to the point of addiction. At conferences of dowsers pendulums are swung to determine whether to order chips or boiled potatoes for lunch. Oracles, however, are not always content with yes/no answers and may well suggest you consider

Dauphinoise, mashed or even no potatoes at all before making your decision.

Jupiter is benevolent, generous and supportive and, fittingly, the planet Jupiter is by far the largest in the solar system. It acts as our protector, its enormous force attracting stray bodies into its orbit where they shatter. The distance between each planet follows a regular pattern but between Jupiter and Mars it is much bigger than one would expect. Between the orbits of the god of war and the god of the thunderbolt is the asteroid belt, a circuit of millions of lumps of rock orbiting the Sun like a planet. This debris is probably the remains of heavenly bodies that Jupiter has destroyed. Some say it includes the planet Phaeton who was killed by Jupiter when he joy-rode his father's Sun-chariot, causing havoc in the universe.

Jupiter, the law-giver, holds ultimate power of life and death. The Sun himself is subject to him and, while the Sun has given his name to our day of rest, it is Jupiter who provides the abundance associated with that day for he not only loves to sow his seeds but to celebrate their fruition. He and Juno are identified with the cornucopia, the horn of plenty which is related to the seventh day and to the month of September when the Sun passes from the sign of Virgo into Libra, the seventh sign. In September we celebrate the harvest and on the sabbath we not only rest and look back at our work to see, like God, 'that it is good', we also eat well, visit relatives and friends, worship and pray. The seventh is a day of celebration, thanksgiving and nourishment. (Or it was until we found ourselves forsaking the aisles of the church for those of the supermarket.)

Jupiter does not suffer fools gladly and, as lord of the thunderbolt, is quick to punish inflated pride, extravagance and deliberate faithlessness. It was he, of course, who struck York Minster with lightning on July 9th 1984 just after the Bishop of Durham raised questions in that building about the nature of God. And it is Jupiter who will reprimand and punish us for the damage we are causing the natural world. Freak floods, hurricanes, volcanic eruptions, earthquakes - Jupiter sends his warnings and retribution through the weather. But, since the chaos we are causing is due to the fact that we have no faith, no sense of cosmic order and no recognition of our place in the universe, there is little chance that we will, en masse, pay heed to the meanings behind such disruptive weather events. We will, instead, try to deal with the holes in the ozone layer by rubbing onto our skins still more lotions from still more plastic bottles or cope with invading deserts by damming still more rivers and so destroy still more eco-systems. We will go on creating material solutions to problems we perceive as only of a material nature. In preparation for the trouble we sense is coming we have built flood barriers and a scheme is even underfoot to construct a gigantic mirror and send it into space in order to reflect the Sun's rays and create artificial daylight in those parts of the Earth that would otherwise be experiencing night. This, we are told, will give rescue teams a better chance to do their work efficiently and have the added bonus of enabling farmers to harvest their crops by night!

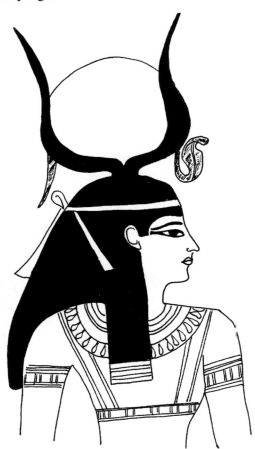

Isis balancing the Solar disc contained within the horns of the Moon.

We have upset the balance not only of nature, but of the seasons, of the atmosphere and of day and night. A giant mirror in space creating extra sunlight at the expense of darkness is a perfect symbol of our concentration on the conscious, the logical or the 'masculine' mind to the detriment of the unconscious, the intuitive, nurturing 'feminine'.

Sun and Moon are counterbalancing forces, their relationship changing with the months, the years, and the cycles of eclipses. They grow weaker and stronger in relation to each other, reaching their perfect balance at full Moon and at the equinoxes. In early Spring, the Golden Measure of the Moon's movements marks the beginning of Easter, the festival of eggs when the mature Sun or son dies in the cradling arms of the Moon or mother and is resurrected anew; in late summer the full Moon marks the harvest, produce of the marriage of male and female, Sun and Moon.

This fundamental seasonal cycle has spawned a wealth of archetypal images, myths, rituals and celebrations. To the Romans, Jupiter and Juno are the fertile, mature couple, overseers of the harvest. To the Christians, the story of the relationship between Sun and Moon is located in the story of Jesus, the Son, and his mother, the Virgin or Moon, and to the Egyptians, the cycle of death and renewal was centred on the king Osiris who descended to Earth from his constellation, and, on departing the physical body to return there at death, fertilised his wife, Isis, the dog-star, Sirius, with the seed that would become the new king, Horus.

Isis is not simply the faithful dog who follows her husband and mourns his loss. She is the inspiration behind all his actions. 'Isis' means 'throne'. This queen is not only the power behind the throne, she is the throne itself. The Egyptian throne, the Goddess Isis, stayed in place over thousands of years and each king that came and went embodied the spirit of Horus, the servant of the culture who perpetually repeats the cycle of death and resurrection.

Isis never needs to take on earthly power because she is the embodiment of a graceful, natural, unforced power. She exists beyond ego and beyond the need herself to implement consciousness. She belongs in the women's room, behind the veil of illusion: 'I am Isis whom no man hath unveiled'. Adjoining the thalamus in the head is what could be understood as Isis herself, the 'pulvinar' or 'cushioned throne of the gods'. Isis is a constant presence, loving and supporting, giving life, witnessing death and guiding the spirit beyond the body. She mourns and regenerates but she is not a public figure. The female, the virgin-mother/ nymph-crone, it would seem from myth, continues to live while the male comes and goes. The feminine is the soul that lives on after the death of the masculine, the conscious, active mind.

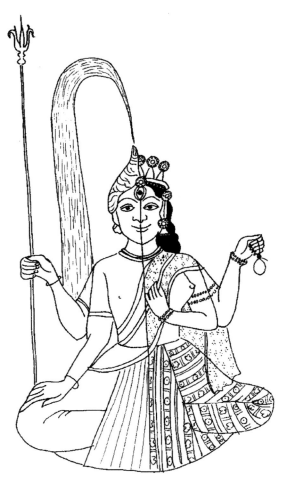

Shiva, uniting the masculine and the feminine, with the Ganges spouting from his head. India. 19th century.

Throughout the world, in countless cultures, the major headdresses of the gods are images of the Sun and Moon. Even Christianity, a monotheistic religion with a consequent lack of variety of divine imagery, shows the halo over all its spiritually evolved beings, forming over the crown of the head when the internal organs of solar and lunar functions - the pineal and pituitary glands - come into balance, when the enlightened being has attained perfection through uniting spiritual and earthly purpose and providing an opening or channel between mortal and immortal life.

The halo appears above the fontanelle. There are several fontanelles on the head, soft pulsing places where, on a young baby, the skull structure has not yet met and rigidified. The largest of them is at the crown. 'Fontanelle' means 'fountain' or 'font' - it is seen on the whale as it rises to the air and the light spouting salt sea water and is depicted on the Hindu god Shiva as the river Ganges shooting from his head.

The crown chakra opens when the other chakras are in balance. It is sometimes known as the 'thousand-petalled lotus', the full blown lily, its fullness reached when innocence has been transformed, through experience, to wisdom. The crown chakra has two parts, an inner and an outer, the inner formed of twelve petals or segments, so reflecting the heart chakra. 'Crown' itself means 'corona', the halo around a heavenly body, and the word corona also refers to the heart - we are familiar with it through the word 'coronary', a heart attack.

Our cronophobic, nympholeptic society chooses to deny the wisdom and power of the crone, just as it refuses to entertain the notion that sometimes men might be weaker than or dependent on women and that consciousness needs the constant support and inspiration of the unconscious. Crone or crown wisdom comes about through the suffering of experience. We all, it would seem, have been meted out our share of suffering but women, according to the Bible, have received an extra large portion in the curse of menstruation and childbirth.

The curse of suffering brings wisdom. Along with one's own birth and death, the act of childbirth is the most demanding task of human life. It is not surprising that over aeons of time sacred practices have developed around death and birth. Vast temples still stand and ancient texts written originally in stone still exist that were constructed to honour the passage from life to death. Undoubtedly, temples and sacred sites have also existed

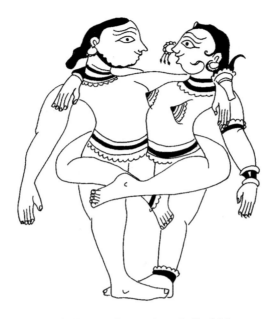

The balance of opposites. India 19th century.

to aid, honour and celebrate the entrance into life. We know of gods and goddesses, like Juno, who, identified with both the apple and the pomegranate, aided the process of conception, gestation and childbirth; we know of sexual practices and rituals which link the sacred and divine with the human form and we have illustrations, writings, sculptures and religious buildings dedicated to a celebration of the symbolic marriage of male and female through sexuality, the balancing of opposites that leads to a transcendence of polarity.

It is often said, with a knowing smirk, that prostitution is the oldest profession. Like mother-in-law jokes, such a remark is of its patriarchal times. If anything can claim to be the oldest profession, it must be midwifery. Prostitution can only exist in cultures in which women are owned and therefore available to be bought and sold. Our culture is one such. However independent, wealthy or free women may feel themselves to be, there is no female centre. The women's room has been destroyed and, with it, the nymphon. What remains of the sacred female temples, the

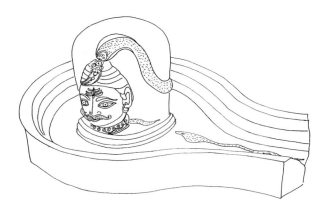

*The sacred union of lingam and yoni decorated with the head of Shiva.
India.*

sanctuaries for the rituals of sex, procreation, gestation, childbirth and
lactation, are tawdry sex shops, brothels, escort agencies and, all over the
world, the sale of young girls for the satisfaction of visiting businessmen
and tourists.

The nymphon was once hung with net and lace spun by the crones or black
widow spiders, and perfumed and prepared by women for sexual practices
which were indistinguishable from spiritual ones. Now that we have
abandoned the thalamus and, with it, the nymphon, women are left seeking
power, along with men, in the outer world. Children, as well as women and
men, are now subject to the 'masculine' 9 to 5 clock, the measurement of
solar time that relates not to inner rhythms but to the market place. The
lunar cycles of women and young children and the seasonal cycles of the
Earth are all but forgotten in our concentration on the conscious and on
daylight. But consciousness is always dependent on the thalamus, day
develops from night, light from dark, life from the source. And there can be
no king without a throne.

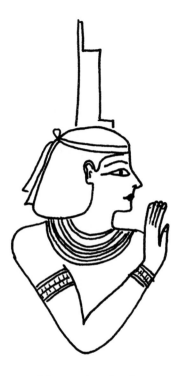

Isis wearing the throne.

A meditation

Sit straight and close your eyes.

Bring your awareness to the heart chakra.

Move up the spine through the centre of the head to the crown chakra just above the head.

Move back down to the heart chakra.

Repeat this movement up and down for three or four minutes, resting momentarily at both the heart and crown chakras.

End at the heart chakra and release contact. Then bring your awareness to the word, 'healing'. Allow what comes forward to take place.

After ten or fifteen minutes, finish by bringing your attention briefly back to the heart chakra.

In place of the word, 'healing', any other word can be used, for instance, 'forgiveness', 'faith', or 'essence'.

Eight
Saturn   The Root

'Man must suffer to be wise.'

Aeschylus

After the harvest comes winter, after the celebration comes the hangover, after expansion comes contraction, after Jupiter comes Saturn, god of restriction, ageing and death.

Until the invention of the telescope, Saturn was thought of as the outermost planet of our system. He was the boundary-maker, dividing the known universe from the unknown, marking the line between infinity and the here and now, providing the framework for the destinies of mortals. He is lord of the finite world, the guardian of the gate, the judge of souls, the time-keeper, overseer of mortality who appears when one's time is up, when the hourglass has run out.

Sun and Moon can be seen as the balance of light and dark within us, providing us with an inner and outer sense of time, Mercury gives us our spinal fluid and nervous system, enabling the body to respond to thought, Venus provides us with flesh and blood, and Mars with the cellular structure. Jupiter sends us sustenance and the faith to give our lives meaning and Saturn gives us the bare bones, the skeleton on which everything else is hung. After all the rest has gone, the bones remain, as part of the Earth itself.

Long-faced Saturn belongs to the grave, in more than one sense. He is the force of gravity itself, holding us to the Earth and confining us to our physical frames and he is the Grim Reaper whose scythe no-one escapes and who sorts the wheat from the chaff. He oversees the law of cause and effect, ensuring that we each receive our due and reap what we have sown.

102

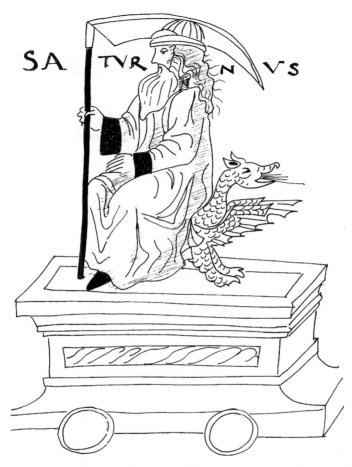

SA TVR N VS

Saturn. Europe. 16th century.

He is old Father Time and the lord of karma, governing the soul's entrance into the mortal body and its departure while ensuring that each incarnation is appropriate to the soul's journey.

Saturn does not excuse mistakes nor turn a blind eye to failings. He is the task-master, akin to the God of the Old Testament, testing, judging and punishing us. While Jupiter is the law-giver, Saturn is the law-enforcer. While Jupiter is lord of abundance, Saturn brings frustration, delay and endless challenge. Saturn demands that one understands oneself and comes to terms with one's limitations. Putting mortals through trial and experience, he gets rid of all that is superfluous. There is no disguise, nowhere to hide from Saturn. He urges us to let go of our illusions, to see reality and to recognise death as the great leveller.

Bringing us down to Earth, he burdens us with responsibilities and duties. He calls for us to come to terms with our lot as human beings, to accept the repetitiveness of work, the discipline of order, to fit into our tradition and heritage, to persist with what has been tried and tested. He is the father and patriarch whose name is carried through the generations and whose word goes.

While Mars is the force that represents the individual will, the wish to assert oneself over nature and make an impact or impression, Saturn gathers, controls and disciplines the generative life force, giving the will duration in time, turning the impulsive sexual energy of Mars into a family or cultural line or tradition. The will is a list of instructions left after death; but Saturn adds to it the testament. A testament, like a testimony or testimonial, is a statement of one's being. It is a way of describing in words what one is and what one believes.

One's beliefs, value and worth lie behind the accumulation and dissemination of one's property and wealth and the 'testament', stemming as it does from the word 'test' and provided by Saturn, the great task master, relates to the testes and to the male hormone, 'testosterone'. Just as the will comes from Mars and the male desire to plant and propagate his seed in Venus and the Earth, so the testament comes from Saturn and the male wish to have his word obeyed and his seed continued throughout the generations. No wonder, when such import is placed on the soft, vulnerable testicles, that men under pressure often appear decidedly 'testy'. The burden that we place on men to produce and perform has, of course, its correspondence in the power that we take away from women: the word testes used to refer also to the female ovaries.

The Word as represented in law and belief is traditionally a male possession. Women have been kept out of the process of law-making and governing, of the priesthood and of the interpretation of the scriptures not as a whim but in a deep-rooted belief that women's words are not to be trusted. Only if you have testicles do you have the right and responsibility to testify: the word 'testes' means both 'testicles' and 'witness'. A man who refuses to testify in court is put under contempt of court but, until very recently, a married woman was not expected or required to testify against her husband and it was considered that a woman's offences were the responsibility of her husband. As late as the 1970s a British high court judge declared that 'women and little boys' should not be trusted because they were renowned for lying. While the husband is subject to the state, the wife is subject to the husband. 'He for God only; she for God in him' (John Milton).

The seeds of Saturn hold the potential of civilisation. They are not only the sperm that can create the future generations but the thoughts that will have repercussions throughout time. They are the carriers of destiny. One inherits one's destiny through the parents and the forefathers. It is through the line that themes unfold and battles are fought. For the Greeks, the fortunes of the individual were inseparable from those of the family House. Women in patriarchal cultures cannot pass on their names since a sur-name, by its very nature, belongs to the 'sire'. The state, the national 'House', is a gathering of families known by their sire names and the males, as representatives of their nation, are required to kill and be killed on its behalf. It is a tragic irony that the only place we see those sire names listed is on each town and village war memorial commemorating the dead whose remains lie anonymously in mass graves on foreign shores.

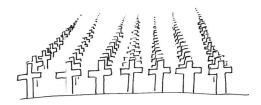

In cultures that believe in reincarnation, karma (the law that posits that each thought, word or action has repercussions that have to be accounted for) is thought to be worked out not only through the lineage but through the individual soul returning time and again to Earth in order to grow through experience towards freedom from the wheel of incarnation. It is said that soul's return to Earth in groups, that we are each connected to others not only for one lifetime but many and that one of the lessons of karma is to release ourselves from the bonds that hold us to others.

When the soul is released from its karma, it is free to choose whether to return into another incarnation or not. When one has reached the level of making real choices, one can see life for what it is, without illusion or desire. One sees that life is a testing ground or threshing floor and full of suffering and, if one chooses to continue to suffer, it is for a purpose. There are countless stories in Buddhism of boddhisatvas, 'realised' beings who return to Earth in order to help others on their journey of development. These are souls who, because of their accumulated compassion and understanding, are able to tolerate all kinds of abuse and suffering and still maintain calm and faith, acting as examples to others.

Freedom from the attachment of earthly desire and illusion and the release from human bonds is freedom from the domain of Saturn who, as Satan, keeps us attached to the ways of the flesh, tempting us with earthly delights, then punishing us for our dependency on them. Man's position on earth is somewhere between the gods and the beasts. He is, perhaps, a descendant of the apes yet blessed or cursed with consciousness, speech and, therefore, responsibility. Man has the ability to tame and control the beasts but must, in turn, obey the gods.

'The beast' is a colloquial term for sexuality or our instinctive nature. It refers to the donkey or ass which is renowned for its lascivious nature and is a form of Satan, the tempter. Like Mars, Saturn was originally a god of agriculture worshipped in the riotous celebrations of the Saturnalia. The devil's purpose is to keep us attached to the plane of earth, the level of gravity and denseness. He seeks to deny us a relationship with God, that is to say, access to our higher natures. The choice is ours but it takes understanding and will power to surmount the temptations of Saturn. He is relentless in meting out suffering and merciless in giving us our due. But it is through him that we eventually learn to take responsibility for ourselves and grow up.

Saturn's orbit hovers between the known and the unknown; through and beyond it we reach freedom. One cannot be truly free until one is detached from Earth and yet one cannot be detached from earth until one has first become established on it. The root chakra, situated just above the base of the spine, provides our relationship to Earth.

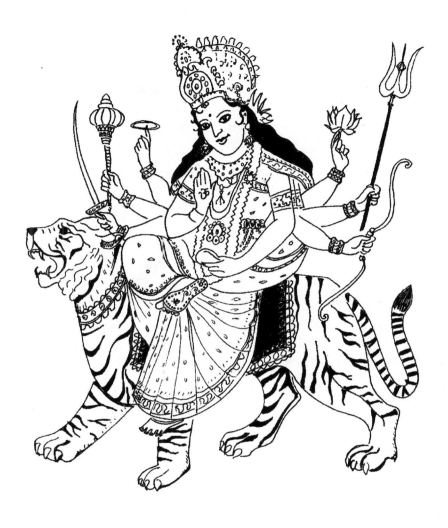

The Hindu goddess Durga whose image is considered so powerful that it is not displayed in many homes. India 20th century.

The root chakra can be found on the spine, its energy extending, a bestial remnant, like a tail towards the Earth. As the lowest, it is the slowest moving chakra. It has four petals or segments and, though it is possible to see or sense these divisions, one can also be pulled into the chakra both on oneself or another person, through a spiral movement. This can occur with any of the chakras since they consist, in fact, of spiral formations, and it can be a very intense movement, taking one into the centre of the chakra and then into what may seem to be another dimension.

The root chakra is associated with the element of earth but its colour is red. The green of the heart is identified with nature and the growth on the crust of the Earth, but the red of the root is related to the fiery centre of the Earth, the fuel that keeps us going but also devours and purifies. Many religions suggest that matter or dross is burned and purified in the lower regions of Earth while the spirit is released heavenward. The fire is, of course, hell and Saturn or Satan is its master taking sinners to eternal damnation or suffering. The damned are those who pursue carnality and the material life at the expense of the spirit.

When the root chakra is strong and energetic it provides a sense of well-being and confidence. One can place one's feet firmly on the ground and feel that one belongs. From such a sense of security one can grow into one's rightful inheritance and fulfil one's purpose. But, where the background is one of confusion, the individual may inherit an inability to make a productive home life from which to feel safe in the world. Low self-esteem, stemming from early insecurity, can influence one's ability to form relationships, to have an effect in the world and may even limit fertility and therefore one's opportunity to plant the seeds of Saturn for the future.

Imbalances at the root cause one to compare oneself with others and create false feelings of success and failure and of superiority and inferiority. The effect may be felt not only personally but culturally. Whole civilisations have been established on the belief that some beings - children, animals, women, blacks, Jews, gypsies, the mentally and physically impaired, etc. - are inferior. The root is the chakra of sexuality and potency. In patriarchal religions, the priesthood is required to deny sexuality while at the same time keeping women from spiritual influence and power.

The sacredness of the female cycle of ovulation, menstruation, gestation, birth, lactation has been so diminished that it is now considered natural to take drugs that alter it and to give birth in hospital, as if being female were a medical condition. The natural protectiveness of a mother towards her children is not only seriously threatened by the way we live but is undermined by the law.

Sadly, there are instances when a mother needs to protect herself and her children not from the world outside so much as from the father or stepfather within the home. Frequently the best the authorities can do is to remove the children from the home. New divorce and custody laws, developed with the unsubstantiated belief that fathers and mothers now share child care, make it increasingly difficult for a mother to protect her children in the case of violence, drug-abuse, and psychological terror.

There once was a time when the exclusion of women from the established religious practices had spiritual significance. But spiritual practice has for centuries in the 'West' been centred only on the outer and the masculine. Women, therefore, have no say in religious beliefs and practices and women's experiences and ways of understanding and, indeed, worshipping have not been validated. The extent to which religious practice involving women and children has been destroyed can be measured by looking at the religious customs that continue around the female cycle. Where are they, one might ask and the question must be followed by other questions: Where is the women's room? And where is the nymphon? And what has happened to the sacred phases of woman: the pupa, the nymph, the spider and the crone?

It is not surprising to find that women's experience has been so thoroughly destroyed. Witch-hunting lasted over three centuries (from the fifteenth to the eighteenth century) and was rampant throughout Europe and America. Millions of women were killed for the crime of being women and thinking and practising in women's ways. In some villages only one woman was left alive, for what purposes one can only morbidly guess at. The ancient respected practice of midwifery (French for midwife is 'sage-femme': wisewoman) was all but destroyed and taken over by the medical profession which was forcefully establishing itself as a closed shop that excluded women practitioners, re-admitting the midwife only in an inferior servicing role to the doctor. Our continuing fear of the witch is reflected in the fact that not only is the massacre of generations of women, children and men as witches virtually ignored in our history books but many schools and libraries now ban the use of children's books that mention the word 'witch'.

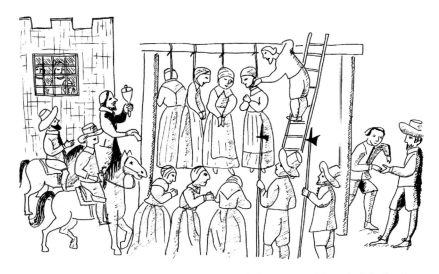

Hanging witches. Newcastle, England. 17th century. The witchfinder is receiving his wages. All the men in the picture are at 'work' (and the women are wearing aprons).

In the face of such denial it is hard to gain an understanding of what 'witchcraft' actually was but it seems from diagrams that have been found marked on floors of Cotswold houses that it was, at least in part, the quest to relate to the divine through symbols and personal reflection rather than the docile acceptance of orthodox teachings.

Our contemporary tendency to expect a woman in childbirth to have as her companion not a mother, sister or wisewoman, but her husband frequently leaves both partners vulnerable and anxious and the childbirth itself the source of disappointment, blame and resentment. Childbirth brings up intense feelings in everyone, women as well as men. Even if there are twelve good fairies present, just one bad one can leave a curse that may take years to undo. In one instance I know, an interesting twist was added to the age-old custom of the anxious father-to-be seeking other female company during his wife's labour. When the labour was well established, the husband disappeared from the wife's bedside and returned some hours later accompanied by his mistress who stayed to watch the birth.

With the disappearance of the wisewoman and the female birthing chamber went the ancient wisdom of healing and prediction derived from a knowledge of the stars, of herbs, of the elements, the weather and so on. To bring it back now must involve the reconstitution of midwifery as a purely female practice respected as the heart of the community. Midwifery is the centre of female work and wisdom, as is what follows it, childcare. There is a fine balance of male and female within our makeup and within the cosmos and it needs to be reflected in the way we organise our society. Equality is meaningless: men and women are not the same any more than the Moon and the Sun are the same. Sun and Moon are in balance only when they are as far apart as they can get, when the Moon is full and opposite the Sun.

The male province has, traditionally, throughout the world, been the outer and the female, the inner. The thalamus has been the heart of all civilisations. The unconscious, therefore, the deep knowing that cannot be subjected to logic, has also been considered sacred and central. Consciousness is the child of the unconscious just as we are all of woman born. Our valuation of the unconscious can be measured by the way we treat women and, through them, children.

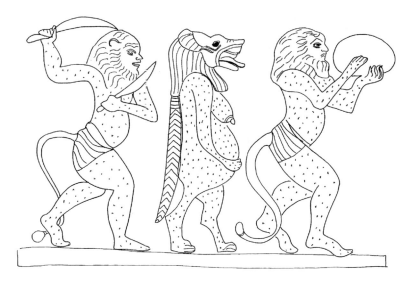

Men dressed as the god of childbirth, Bes, dancing round the pregnant goddess, Taueret. Greek.

In religious cultures where the emphasis is on the outer, 'masculine' form of religious practice to the detriment or even exclusion of the inner, 'feminine' form, belief is dictated by outer authority. It is not only impossible but sacrilegious to find one's own inner truths and beliefs. One has to toe the spiritual line which comes direct from an asexual male god through his asexual male priests and then to the people. Sexuality and spirituality have not always been separated as they are in our western cultures today. In practising them as one, women went through their transformations from pupa to pia mater to arachnoid mater to crone with awareness and understanding, celebrating their ability not only to create and nurture life but to use their natural intuition and wisdom to weave the web of fate.

The spider in mythology weaves the world into being, she is responsible for life and death and for fate itself. She makes the web, the very stuff of life, the illusory net on which all life is hung. She is associated with the number eight, the symbol of the hour-glass that can be perpetually turned upside-down as one cycle of time ends and another is begun. On its side, the figure eight makes the symbol for infinity and, as two squares, one shown as a diamond outside the other, eight provided the alchemists with a diagram that contained all possible variations of existence.

Eight belongs not only to the spider but to the crab and octopus, all images of the Great Mother. The octopus has many arms, like the Hindu gods and goddesses whose hands each carry a different symbol, showing their many aspects. Eight represents a contented stability which, nonetheless, contains all possibilities. The solar system with Saturn as its boundary contains eight bodies (including the earth); within its boundaries is everything we need for earthly existence. But beyond Saturn lies a greater freedom, a possibility of evolution beyond what is tried and tested to a brave new world.

A grounding exercise

.   Stand comfortably balanced with feet apart, in line with your hips.

Close your eyes. Bring your awareness to the pineal chakra on the forehead.

Then come down the front of the body to the hara area.

Take your awareness down the right leg to beneath the foot and, as you do so, gradually move all your weight onto that foot.
Bring your awareness across to beneath the left foot and, as you do so, place all your weight on that foot.

Come up the left leg to the hara area while balancing the weight evenly again.

From the hara area, travel back down the right leg as before.

Continue with this triangular formation for ten minutes.

To finish, come back up the body from the hara area to the pineal chakra.

Nine
Uranus The Mental Aura

'I am he as you are he as you are me and we are all together'.
Lennon and McCartney

Following hot on the heels of the discovery that the Sun, not the Earth, was at the centre of our planetary system, came the discovery that Saturn did not, after all, mark the boundary. There were other planets beyond his orbit, planets that could only be seen with the aid of the newly-invented telescope. The first to be found was Uranus.

To shift one's belief that the square plane of Earth is at the centre of a system bounded by the great patriarch, Saturn, to an understanding that the Earth is actually a tiny round ball spinning round a massive central Sun and that the solar system extends way into the deep beyond and holds within it other, as yet undiscovered, mysterious and, possibly, sinister forces is not an easy thing to do. No wonder those who suggested such a radical reappraisal of the world picture were condemned as heretics. They were not only challenging the beliefs of many hundreds of years, they were challenging Saturn's order and authority itself.

While the Earth is the planet of tension and struggle, the Sun is the place of individuality, joy, creativity and the energy that William Blake described as perpetual delight. To see one's own creative impulses at the centre of the universe in place of the limitations of duty and responsibility and to let go of the sense of outer boundary in favour of limitless possibility is to make oneself answerable only to one's own inner Sun, one's own soul.

The new understanding of the nature of the universe entailed not only a reappraisal of the motions of physical celestial bodies. The planets were gods that ruled our individual and collective lives. As they moved through their orbits they, themselves, underwent constant shifts of alignment and relationship with each other. The Earth provided the square plane on which the struggle of life took place and Saturn provided the cube that contained everything. There was no escape from such a prison and those who attempted to go beyond the patriarchal order whether by witchcraft, magic, theological challenge or political revolt were punished in a most Saturnian way.

The huge shift in the world picture that took place during the periods we know as the Renaissance and Enlightenment enabled an assertion of self against state, church and all other hierarchies. The god of individuality and creativity could now be found within, at the centre of each person and there was no longer any need to stay within the bounds of inherited beliefs.

Uranus was discovered on March 13th 1781, a time when kings were challenged and even beheaded and democracies established, when New Worlds were founded, when countless inventions made it possible for individuals to alter their ways of working, travelling and living. Uranus

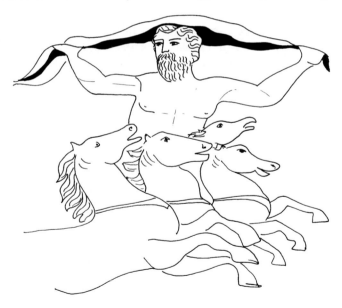

Uranus holding up the sky.

himself became identified with freedom of thought, with radical beliefs and movements that could challenge the existing order and bring into being the creativity of the individual, original mind. As god of heaven, Uranus belongs to the blue beyond, the place of aspiration, dreams, hopes and wishes, a place where the mind can soar and the spirit can fly beyond the limits of the physical form.

Though Uranus is the herald of democracy, freedom and fraternity, the killer of kings and the liberator of individuality, he, himself, is a patriarch. He is married to Mother Earth, Gaia, and at first resided within her. It was only with an almighty struggle (of the kind that many of us experience when separating from our mothers) that he managed to get free of her and set himself way beyond her dominion. But his relationship with Gaia thrives to this day and all that is born of Earth is engendered by the god of Heaven.

And, though we think of Saturn as the ultimate patriarch, stickler for order and duty and minding your p's and q's, he himself was once a revolutionary upstart. Saturn only came to power through the overthrow of his father, Uranus, and he did this in a way that was symbolic of Saturn's authority - he cut off his father's testicles and threw them into the sea. In order to establish the line of his own seed, his word or testament, he had to dispose of his father's. The seed of Uranus is highly productive. He is not only

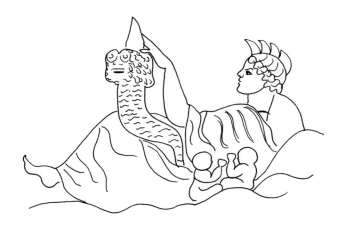

Gaia with some of her children.

father of all that is produced by Mother Earth, but from the union of his testicles with the other Great Mother, the Sea, the Mere or Mer, Venus arose from the surface of the ocean shrouded in the mists of illusion. Venus, mother of humanity, is daughter of Uranus, god of heaven.

To understand the nature of Uranus is to put Saturn in his place as the father of earthly traditions and mores and to find the possibility of shedding

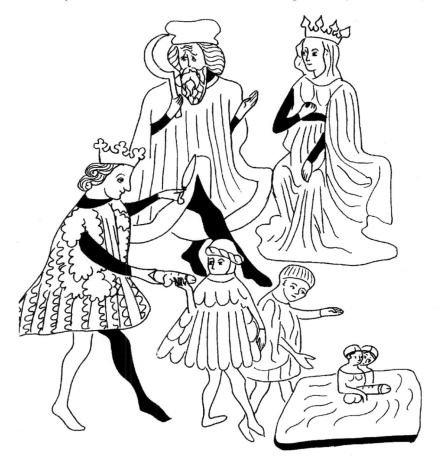

Jupiter passes the castrated genitals of his father, Saturn, to join those of his grandfather, Uranus. Europe 15th century.

inherited systems of belief to reach towards one's own interpretation or knowledge of the universe both within and without. But this is a dangerous enterprise. Uranus is volatile. Since he lies beyond the influence of Saturn, he is not subject to the normal rules and regulations. To tamper irresponsibly with the energies of Uranus is to wreak havoc and destruction on Earth.

Uranus, detached from earthly bonds and the earthly pull of gravity, is of the head and the number nine. While six is the number of sex, procreation and the cellular structure, nine is the number of mind, thought and genius. Nine is the limit, the peak - and the sister of Uranus, Urania, is goddess of the mountains and of astronomy. If you multiply nine by any number and add the resulting digits the total will always be nine. For instance: three times nine makes twenty-seven; add two and seven and you get nine. Or: 634 times 9 makes 5706; 5+7+0+6=18; 1+8=9. Nine is a full-stop or a summit; you can go no further. All you can do is start again with nought. Nine is definitive, repetitive and predictable. Beyond gambling or guesswork, it is the number of the godhead, almighty and unchanging.

Six and nine fit together like peas in a pod. Lying down, 6 and 9 form the zodiacal sign of Cancer, the crab or Great Mother, the unconscious universe before division occurred. Uranus and Gaia need each other. They are the forces of evolution, the constant interchange of spirit and matter that allows growth and development. In order for the marriage of Uranus and Gaia to be the productive relationship it is, the male had to detach himself from the female and each partner has to have their own dominion; only then can they meet as polar opposites and produce their manifold offspring. The Egyptians knew this too. Although their sky was female, represented by the goddess Nut whose beautiful slim body arches over the world and is studded with stars, and their Earth was male, represented by Nut's brother, Geb, it was still essential to them that Heaven and Earth maintained their separate realms.

Six and nine make the ancient symbol of yin and yang, the philosophy that proposes that everything in existence is subject to polarity. The black head of one tadpole contains a white eye and the white head of the other contains a black one.

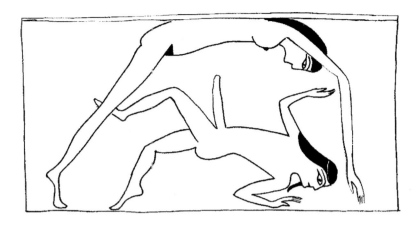

Nut and Geb. Eygpt.

Through the eye, it is implied, the one changes into the other; black becomes white and white, black. The symbol shows the two in perfect balance but the balance cannot last. When fullness is reached, decline occurs; one thing waxes while another wanes, day becomes night and night, day, the strong becomes weak and the weak, strong. This is the principle behind the workings of the ancient Chinese book of divination, the I Ching, in which the hexagrams are formed of lines signified by the numbers 6, 7, 8 and 9. It is the lines made by the numbers 6 and 9 that give way into their opposites and so cause the creation of a new hexagram and another oracle.

Where yin and yang is a flourishing concept so, inevitably, is a belief in reincarnation. The yin and yang tadpoles exist within a circle, a chakra, the wheel of life itself that goes on turning while lives come and go. The concept of yin and yang is not confined to the Chinese. Similar beliefs in the creative pull of opposing forces can be found all over the world.

Christianity, which was at first a radical challenge to existing authorities, propounding the importance of each person finding their own way to a meeting with the divine, held to the notion of reincarnation until the Second Council of Constantinople in 553 AD when the belief became a punishable heresy.

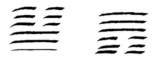

'Peace' becomes 'Standstill'.

The first shall be last and the last, first. When one thing becomes too full it gives way to its opposite. This, it would seem, is a universal law. If, over time, the male becomes female and the female, male, the black becomes white and the white, black, the oppressed becomes the oppressor and the oppressor the oppressed, then how you treat others is inseparable from how you treat yourself.

The Uranian challenge is to create something new, fresh and original that will not decay into the very conditions from which it has escaped. It is the challenge that revolutionaries rarely succeed in meeting, as the initial positive energy of the revolution rigidifies into something as terrible as what preceded or inspired it. The danger that Uranus poses is of losing contact with the Earth, of allowing thought to dictate, of forsaking heart and common sense in favour of dogma and the pursuit of ideas for their own sake.

Until the great revolutions of our age it had been generally assumed that the rule of kings was a natural, or divine, one. In ancient Egypt or China, for example, the kingdom remained much the same for thousands of years. And still, in the West today, we organise animals, plants and the natural world into 'kingdoms'.

A kingdom has an inbuilt order and structure. It has a hierarchy and each stratum within it knows its place. To step beyond the bounds of Saturn and overthrow the natural order is to upset the hierarchical balance. The discovery of Uranus has been synchronous not only with the radical reappraisal of human systems of government but with human interference in the established order within the natural world. Frankenstein's monster, an image created by Mary Shelley just after the French revolution and the discovery of Uranus, has been let loose on the world. The monster is not of woman born but is the product of the number 9, the head without the nurturing receptacle of the number 6. The scientific mind has assumed precedence over all other ways of understanding and we are without a spiritual value system to hold it back or contain it.

Only a hundred years ago American Indians were warning 'civilised' man of the dangers inherent in assuming that one could possess the land. We now not only own land and alter it and all that lives on it according to our own wants, we also interfere with the very structure of nature. It is as impossible to control genetic engineering as it was to control the single-minded ambition to split the atom. The mind is no longer subject to spiritual guidance or to the needs of the earth herself; in other words, the forces of Uranus are no longer subject to Gaia and have, indeed, been let loose to cause havoc and destruction within her. Much of what we call science, harnessed as it is to financial gain and, therefore, to exploitation, is little more than delinquency.

Nuclear waste that is the result of the misuse of uranium threatens the entire world. In parts of what was once the Soviet Empire, nuclear reactors of the same style of the one that leaked in Chernobyl in 1986 are leaking regularly. Children in Sofia in Bulgaria have faces covered with sores that will not heal.

We know that nuclear damage causes distortions in the gene structure of future generations. A portion of the North Sea is now nicknamed 'the hospital ward' by fishermen because the fish there suffer from obscene malformities due to the dumping of waste. The fish is the symbol of Christ: its huge pineal gland in its vesica-shaped body could be represented like this, the union of solar and lunar principles, the Son within his Mother:

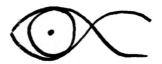

The American Indians, apparently, knew of the existence of Uranus which can just be detected with the naked eye. Amongst their many wise sayings was the reminder that anything we do today has repercussions for another seven generations. Little did they know what was to come - within a couple of generations of the mass slaughter of the native American people and animals, the atom was split, its tests taking place on Indian sacred ground, leaving damage that will last for many thousands of generations.

Scientific discoveries can only be beneficial when linked to real human need and only when in line with the forces of nature. Real progress comes from the marriage of Gaia and Uranus, the interchange of feeling and thought, the honouring of both matter and spirit. Those revolutionaries who, like Mahatma Gandhi, Nelson Mandela or Martin Luther King, make a lasting impact do so by the example of their own enlightening presence, not by force but by transcending the opposing factions and opening new possibilities for the future. To transcend opposition is to reach a state of balance where not only mind and body are united but the two hemispheres of the brain reach a blend. When left and right, logic and intuition blend, the way is opened for enlightenment to take place.

Enlightenment is the fourth stage in the process of meditation. The first is *concentration*, the focus of attention; then comes *meditation* itself, the movement away from the conscious mind into a deeper state of awareness. This is followed by *contemplation* when a point, image, symbol or shape may lead one into a reality beyond that which we associate with the Earth. And, finally, one reaches *illumination* or *enlightenment*.

Enlightenment occurs when sound and light meet. Sound and light are carried through the senses of hearing and sight and the place where the optical and auditory nerves meet is the centre of the head, behind the thalamus. The physical senses are only a portion of our ability to perceive the world. What we see, hear, touch, smell and taste is only a limited range of all that influences us. It is extremely common for people to see and hear clairvoyantly and clairaudiantly and in the practice of meditation and healing a finer attunement to smell, taste and touch is also developed.

To sense clearly is to penetrate the physical to the energy that exists both within the physical and beyond it. To ignore or deny the existence of the energy field or aura is to leave ourselves open to untold damage. In taking the aura for granted, we affect or pollute it without allowing ourselves the

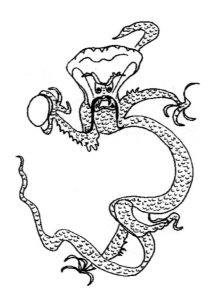

A Chinese dragon holds the pearl of enlightenment.

means to cleanse it. We then become aware of it only when it shows itself as ailing - as has happened with the ozone layer and atmosphere around the earth.

If we had no name for an elbow or an ankle or a dimple, we would rarely come across the need to identify them. When you do not know the name for vetch or loosestrife or cranesbill you tend not to see the plants. And so it is with the aura. Though we think of it, if we think of it at all, as invisible, it is surprising how much of it we can become aware of once we know it is there. The aura, like any territory, can be mapped and has, of course, been depicted throughout the centuries in the art of all cultures. Within its definite boundaries are specific points and streams. The most commonly illustrated part of the aura is the Mental Aura.

The Mental Aura forms a yellow oval shape around the head. It has a fixed rim but, in a person who has developed their awareness and concentration, the inner part of the aura can be seen to extend beyond the outer rim.

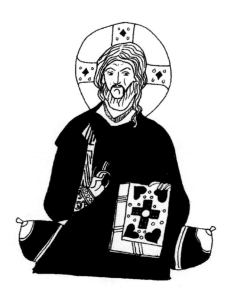

Christ with the cross within the halo.

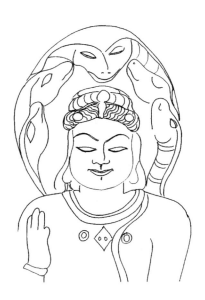

Nagas, divine snakes.

The apex of the mental aura is the Individuality, Soul or Essence Point. It is situated about eighteen inches, or half a metre, above the crown of the head and can be surprisingly easy to contact. The rim of the Mental Aura descends from the Individuality Point all round the head and comes into the chakra system through a point on the edge of each shoulder, tapering into the heart chakra.

There are six entrances to the centre of the head. From above, one can enter through the crown chakra, from below through the thyroid chakra and the neck. From the front the pineal can draw one inside and at the back the medulla provides access. (See chapter 10). And either side of the head just above the ears are the ear streams.

Each ear stream is formed of a spiral which spreads out in a cone shape and extends way beyond the side of the head. The more awareness a person develops, the looser the spirals become. In someone who relies on borrowed patterns of thinking and has not developed their own beliefs the ear streams are held densely, close to the head.

It is not only the ear streams but the ear itself that is formed of a spiral shape. Spirals carry sound or vibration - a mechanical clock sounds the hour through the motion of a gong on a metal spiral. The inner ear is called the cochlea or 'sea-snail'. The sea-snail or 'nautilus' is considered to be the perfect or 'golden' spiral, which is a basic form in sacred geometry. The

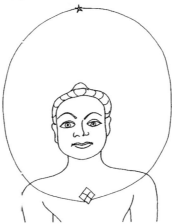

The mental aura.

cochlea are situated either side of the third ventricle, the sea in the head whose tides you can hear if you hold a spiral shell to the ear.

The ear is the first organ formed in the developing foetus and is itself foetal shaped. Sperm and egg are attracted to each other through the medium of sound. All over the world the word OM is celebrated as the first sound, the call that means 'I am' and suggests the awakening of consciousness. It refers to the beginning and the end, providing the first two letters of 'omphalos' which means 'umbilicus' or 'navel', the spiral through which we absorb our first nourishment and which links us to our source and the first two letters of 'omega', the end of all things.

If conception is a big bang, a fusion, an explosion of light and sound, then so is enlightenment, a process that occurs when light and sound meet in the thalamus causing a sudden awakening, a sense of complete understanding or realisation. While conception takes place when sperm and egg, male and female, meet in the womb, enlightenment occurs when the forces of logic and intuition, male and female, fuse in the salt waters of the centre of the head.

Male and female, consciousness and the unconscious, combine their creative powers within the feminine, the unconscious, the womb, the waters of the deep. Though enlightenment takes place in the head, it is not limited to the brain. In enlightenment one is beyond thought and emotion, in a place where one does not think but 'knows'. This is the state of gnosticism when the question of belief is no longer relevant. As Carl Jung said when asked if he believed in God: 'I do not believe; I know'.

Knowledge in ancient times was passed on not as it is today in our secular society as something separate, to be understood only with the conscious brain. The imparting of knowledge was inseparable from experience. Experience and learning give the means to know for oneself. Guarding the frontal conscious brain are the temples. Once, all learning, culture, healing and even business and politics took place in relation to the temples. It was recognised that all thought and all action is dependent on the source, that everything that passes through the brain and the body stems ultimately from the thalamus.

An exercise

Make contact with the heart chakra.

Move from there up through the neck, the centre of the head, out at the crown chakra and up to the Individuality Point. The Individuality Point is situated about half a metre or eighteen inches above the head.

Come down either side of the head in the mental aura, and through the shoulder points back to the heart chakra. The shoulder points are situated on the very edge of each shoulder.

Rest at the heart chakra and repeat.

Finish after ten or fifteen minutes at the heart chakra.

Ten
Pluto   The Medulla

> '*Now when the bardo of the moment before death dawns upon me,*
> *I will abandon all grasping, yearning and attachment, ...*
> *As I leave this compound body of flesh and blood*
> *I will know it to be a transitory illusion*'.
>
> The Tibetan Book of the Dead

Pluto is generally considered to be the outermost planet in the solar system and was the most recently discovered. But, at the moment, it is actually closer to us and, therefore, to the Sun, than is Neptune. Pluto was originally named 'Planet X' by its discoverer, Peercival Lowell, who posited its existence on the assumption that another planet must be contributing to the eccentric orbit of Neptune. When actually seen in 1930, the planet and its path tallied neatly with what had been predicted. In fact, Pluto could have been discovered a lot earlier. It showed up in an early space photograph at the end of the last century but, because no-one was looking for it, no-one saw it.

Such obscurity appears to be an attribute of Pluto whose realm is only experienced in states beyond consciousness. The unrecognised photographic image was taken at the same time that the study of the subconscious was taking form, and the eventual discovery of Pluto occurred at a time when tyrannical dictatorships were gripping much of the world, the following years bringing to light the evil of which humanity is capable. Pluto rules the deepest darkest areas of our beings, his dominion lies well below the rational mind and yet his power is frequently ignored or even denied recognition. It is more comfortable not to know about the underworld and Pluto also rules our tendency to turn a blind eye, our strong and deluded impulse to pretend there is nothing amiss.

Since 1969 Pluto has been within the orbit of Neptune and will stay there until 2009. In 1989 it reached perihelion, that is to say, it came as close as it ever gets to the Sun. The planet takes 282 years to orbit the Sun and perihelion will not occur again until 2217. 1989 coincided with the Chinese year of the snake, creature of the Underworld and identified with the fall; and with the Western year of the pearl, the precious stone of death and conception. 1989 was the year that the Berlin wall came down and the Soviet Empire collapsed and the year that Nelson Mandela was released from jail. The legacies of Hitler and Stalin and the system of apartheid reached a moment of change. Secrets were exposed and long-held grievances and hatreds surfaced. This period while Pluto is as close as it gets to us, gives us, perhaps, a better chance than ever to understand the province of Pluto, to examine both the individual and the mass unconscious. It is as though Pluto, during the short period that it is this side of Neptune's orbit, is offering us the opportunity to explore the Underworld.

There are countless stories about the Underworld. When dissociated from Hell, the terrifying place of perpetual torment, the Underworld is almost a place of comfort, a retreat, a place of hibernation, redolent of the sweet melancholy of loss. In reaching the Underworld, one may meet up with

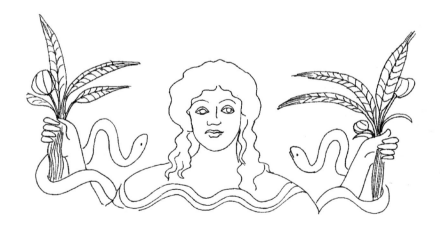

Demeter (or Ceres), goddess of the harvest.

one's fears but also with one's soul, one's loved-one, one's animus or
anima.

One of the best known of those who have descended into the Underworld is
Persephone, daughter of Ceres, goddess of the corn and harvest, and niece
of Hades, the Greek counterpart of Pluto, of Poseidon (the Greek Neptune)
and of Zeus (Jupiter). (The Greek name for Persephone is Kore which
means not only 'maiden' and 'bride' but 'the pupil of the eye'.) Persephone
was innocently playing in a field of narcissi when the ground opened
revealing a field of lilies and Uncle Hades drew her down to his domain
where he seduced her. She fell in love with him and became his wife,
Queen of the Underworld. Through the persuasion of Ceres, Hades
eventually agreed to allow Persephone to return to the Earth for six months
(some say three months and some say nine) of each year. But, because she
had tasted the seeds of the pomegranate or many-seeded apple, the
forbidden fruit, Persephone had to descend again to the Underworld each
autumn.

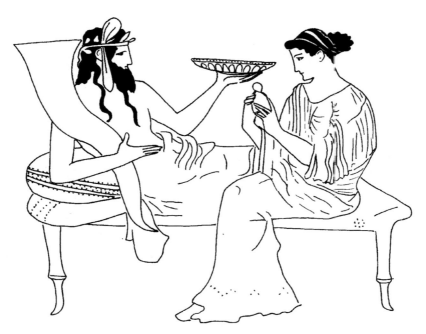

Pluto and Persephone

Persephone's is a story of death and regeneration, echoing that of the Fall, and of the feminine passage from one state of being to another. Persephone, a prototype Lolita, wanders away from her mother to the field of narcissi, the plant of the nymph, of self-awareness and vanity and from there enters the field of lilies, the flower of virginity and death. Young, beautiful, innocent and carefree, she is trapped by the King of the Underworld, and, through sexual knowledge, becomes his queen. The pupa turns into the nymph who in turn is transformed into the crone, queen or wise woman.

The story of Persephone links the female cycle with that of the natural world and, through the figures of Ceres and Hades, shows the fertile relationship between summer and winter, life and death, light and dark, south and north. 'Persephone' means 'the bringer of the light' and she is related to the swallow, the bird that travels between the hemispheres, heralding the approach of summer, the bird described in the Egyptian 'Book of the Dead' as carrying the soul from the dead body to the Sun.

It is not only a tale of transformation, love and regeneration but of incest, rape and the struggle for custody. Though it is agreed that Persephone should return to her uncle/husband each year and, though she loves and needs him and swells into her role as Queen of the Underworld, it is essential that she ascend to her mother, the fruitful Earth, in order to give birth and to celebrate the harvest. The daughter needs the mother just as the mother needs the daughter. When that relationship is interrupted, when the wise older woman is not allowed to guide and nurture the younger, the whole of nature comes under threat.

Pluto absorbs and devours what is no longer purposeful on Earth but, for human beings, that can mean loss, grief and bereavement. The movement from Earth to Underworld and back entails a rite of passage in which the entrance and exit are crucial. Pluto is the door, the gate, the curtain and the veil. Access is only given when the time is right.

While Saturn is the scythe that cuts down the harvest, Pluto gathers the debris, the detritus, the waste and fromit, and makes the manure that feeds the growing seed. The transformation that Pluto produces takes place in dark and secret places. He rules sewers, the colon, the witches brew, the womb, caves, dungeons and orifices. Though he is the destroyer, Pluto serves the purpose of clearing space for the new. Through the endlessly repeated cycle of destruction and resurrection, decay and purification, one attains wisdom. It is in Pluto's domain beneath the ground that precious stones and jewels are formed over aeons.

Darkness is essential for transformation. If you expose the growing form too early, you abort it. If you do not get enough sleep you go mad. Pluto demands that we trust natural processes, that we surrender to the unknown and that we do not interfere with what nature has decreed. In darkness one is free of the body, of the physical senses and is, therefore, closer to one's own soul. The soul is one's inmost being but is also one's other half, the true self for which one is constantly yearning and searching. For men, it is the anima, or female inspirational presence and for women it is the animus, the potent male power that one senses within oneself and may see at times reflected in real human beings. Marriage is an attempt to pledge union with one's soul, to find through commitment to another being of the opposite sex the means to transcend oneself.

Marriage can be represented by the number 10. The upright and the circle are the finger and the ring. They are the union of opposites: logic and intuition, time and space, male and female, lingam and yoni, consciousness and the unconscious. 1 is identity, 0 is embrace. 1 is the individual, 0 is the birth canal and the tunnel of death. 1 is being, 0 is non-being. 1 is the spine, 0 is the halo or aura. 1 and 0 form the maypole, the dance of life; they are the stick and the hoop, creating movement and progression. They are the binary system, the basis of all computing, and they are the particle and the wave: if you choose one you exclude the other, choose being and you exclude non-being, choose non-being and you exclude being.

Ten is the beginning of a new cycle. Infinite noughts can be added to ten, turning the marriage of one and nothing into a harem. Millions and billions, trillions and zillions trip off the tongue and mean 'lots'. The Taoist 'ten thousand things' are the whole of creation.

Our ten fingers and ten toes, bring together the two fives, two halves, left and right. Together, the two hands form a clasp like that of the scallop that enclosed Venus and of the oyster that produces the pearl. Open them and they become a bowl or a cup, an offering. They can give and take, they can share. The pearl is the symbol of marriage, of conception and of death, traditionally given by the husband to the wife to ensure and celebrate fertility. We pass through the pearly gates when we die but the pearl is also the symbol of the new life formed from the union of opposites.

132

In the marriage ceremony, the united couple walk back down the aisle arm in arm. The groom has his right hand free with which to hold his sword while the bride has her left arm free with which to cradle the baby. The right hand is the outgoing one, the one with which we act decisively. The left is the inward one, steadying, balancing, holding. The right flails purposelessly without the left and the left is undirected without the right. Left represents our destiny and right our choices.

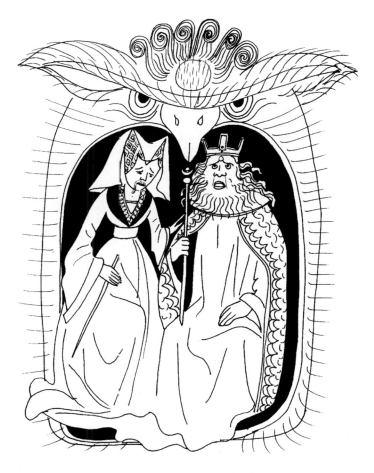

Persephone as Crone with Pluto

The left side of the body is governed by the right side of the brain and vice versa. The two hemispheres of the brain are clearly defined separate entities divided by a channel. The nerves from each side of the brain cross to the opposite side of the body at the medulla oblongata (meaning 'long marrow') which is situated deep in the primitive ancient brain where the top of the spine meets the skull at the cerebellum or Tree of Life.

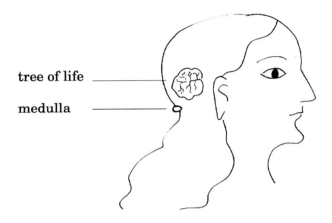

tree of life

medulla

The medulla is a place of great power, opening to dimensions beyond our material world and releasing used energy as it moves up the spine into the head. As energy passes up the spine it feeds numerous emotions, from self-doubt through anger to fear, grief and disappointment. In the recesses of the brain may be buried all kinds of old grievances, resentments and jealousies. The medulla, situated between head and spine or mind and body can act as a link between thought and emotion and, like the exhaust of a car, may discharge the poisonous gases of stale emotions and release the mind from the traumas of the past. Or it may become blocked with unresolved thoughts and emotions forming an obstacle like a boulder at the entrance to a cave and leaving the poison to damage the body.

Energy passes to and fro between the body and its world in many forms, some of them tangible like tears, sweat, saliva, faeces, and food; some less so, like sound, vision and speech, and others still more ethereal, like dream images and psychic perceptions. The medulla is where we let go of our conscious selves. Letting go, though essential for health, can be one of the most difficult things to do. It brings one into the unknown, and can be compared to the descent into the Underworld but only through entering the darkness can one find the light that will take one through to another phase. In the process of death, energy leaves the body just above the medulla and passes along the 'silver cord' referred to in the Bible.

Ten provides the balance of left and right and completes the human being. But the individual being is still only half a polarity, either male or female. The human form has five points and makes a star with its legs, arms and head. The star symbolises an individual fate but the marriage union, for better or worse, joins two fates and establishes a lineage, a family destiny. Two stars united may produce a perfect binary system or the strife of crossed destinies.

In Roman numerals, ten is represented as a cross. All roads lead to Rome and the X is four arrowheads pointing to the centre. The X is the end of a journey and the beginning. It is Planet X, the place of transformation. The cross is a marker, for either good or bad. It marks a destiny, a buried treasure, a secret, it is the sign on the door of dwellings that harbour the plague, it marks trees destined to be felled, it is the crossbones, an intimation of death. Crossed fingers make the wish that destiny will bring good fortune. A finger laid across the lips asks for secrecy and silence. A cross on a letter is a seal and a kiss and a kiss can be for life, for death or for transformation.

When the princess kisses the frog he turns into a prince, when the prince kisses the Sleeping Beauty she wakes into womanhood, when Beauty kisses the Beast his heart is touched and he gains humanity, when Persephone kisses Hades a marriage takes place between life and death.

Sex, like gestation, needs privacy and darkness. The union of oneself with one's soul can only take place beyond consciousness and the light of day. The myths related to Pluto suggest that to see your lover, to expose your soul to the light of day, is to lose him or her.

Psyche was visited every night by her lover, Amor (son of Venus), and transported in the darkness to places of ecstasy but she had to agree never to

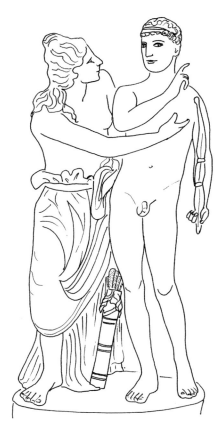

Psyche and Amor

try to look at him and, when she broke the promise, oil from her lamp spluttered on her lover and she lost him.

The tale of Orpheus is even sadder. He lost his lover, Eurydice, when she was bitten by a snake but he managed, and this is something very few of the living can do, to enter the realm of the dead and to beg Hades to give him back his beloved. Hades is not one to give way to special pleading but eventually he agreed, though only on condition that Orpheus did not look back at his lover while leading her up to the world of the living. When, just as he reached the gateway to earth where light was flooding into the Underworld, Orpheus could resist no longer and turned back, Eurydice was lost forever.

Orpheus entered the Underworld through a mirror; in other words, like Narcissus, the iris, and like Persephone, he entered his own reflection to find his soul. The Underworld takes us deeper into ourselves into areas that defy and erode the conscious, rational mind. To go into the Underworld and back can destroy the balance of the mind and poor Orpheus spent the rest of his days a mad recluse, playing his lute to the trees. The lover, the soul, must remain symbolically unseen. Love grows through trusting to intangible forces. The lover is both soul and muse informing and inspiring consciousness to action. Anonymity adds an extra erotic dimension: that is part of the reason that women remain in much of the world behind veils and closed doors.

An Egyptian friend tells me that in Cairo university the women are not permitted to attend the lectures with the men so they watch the lecturers on a television screen in a separate room where they take off their chowdahs and lie around in their jeans and T-shirts chewing gum. There are advantages, she tells me, to the chowdah. If you want an illicit affair it can be quite easily arranged and you have the protection of anonymity. Since women cannot walk around unprotected and are not permitted to drive, a line of cars driven by men is to be found each evening waiting outside the university much as at 3.30 in England the streets outside schools are blocked with mothers waiting in cars for their children. It is not unheard of for a veiled woman, who can see but not be seen, to choose another car to enter and for the car to be seen steaming off into the distance. The frisson of the masked ball is a daily event in Cairo.

Though Pluto would seem to be beyond the codes and rules of Earth, through exposing what is hidden and corrupt he brings about the call for justice. The colon is related to the sense of sight and to the eyes. In clearing waste from this most emotionally sensitive area, we clear ourselves of what may have caused us to turn a blind eye to detrimental or unhealthy situations. Pluto prompts us to action when we realise that to continue to live in a state of corruption or confusion is to be an agent of it. The action we then take may appear to others to be unreasonable or even destructive, but Pluto destroys and discards in order to make way for new growth.

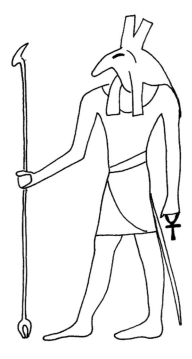

Seth. Egypt.

Every religion has its dark gods which, as long as we do not understand them, remain threatening, anarchic forces. Taming the dragon is an age-old task. The Egyptians showed a simple and effective method: when you meet a monster coming towards you, grip its neck in the fork of your stick (or 'was sceptre') and turn its head around so that it walks in future by your side, as your protection. Their dark dog-like god, Seth, is both a threat to and an ally of the Sun and his enormous power can be harnessed for the good and the light.

Dark gods that draw us into the Underworld allow us to meet our souls, known in Greek as the 'anima', a word closely associated with 'animal'. Many of the Egyptian gods were, in fact, animals or represented as animal heads on human bodies. While the Christian church has decided that animals do not have souls, the Egyptians believed that not only were animals gods but that they could instruct and guide us. To be visited and instructed by a god is, of course, an honour and an awesome event. The Egyptians knew it as the 'ba', the process by which a particular god would, through blending with the soul of a person, appear to them to guide and direct them.

In gaining a god 'on one's side', one develops the strength to defy scepticism and hostility and, like Joan of Arc, Florence Nightingale, Deitrich Bonhoeffer and countless others who have heard the 'calling', the voice of God, to turn adversity to personal advantage and to gain ever greater determination and power from the experience of rejection and betrayal.

The age of Uranus made possible the social and industrial revolutions and the call for democracy. The age of Pluto took us a step beyond, its discovery coinciding with the rise of fascism and the totalitarian state. But Communism in Eastern Europe and National Socialism in Germany in the 1930's could only have come into being through the earlier overthrow of inherited forms of government. The realisation that the power of kings could be abolished and replaced by the 'rights of man' had led naturally to women also demanding rights and Mary Wollstonecroft, mother of Mary Shelley, wrote her famous book on the rights of woman at the time of the French Revolution.

It is curious that, though we live in what we like to call a democracy, we do not honour those who fought for it. Statues to Tom Paine, author of one of the most influential books in the English language, *The Rights of Man*, or to Mary Wollstonecroft are thin on the ground and their books are not read in schools. Caroline Norton, indefatigable Victorian campaigner on behalf of women to keep their children on divorce, is all but forgotten. In forgetting our history, we expose ourselves to the danger of reversal and betrayal. Rights that have been won over years of struggle can be abolished at the stroke of a pen.

Without our noticing, the right of divorced women to keep their children has been subtly eroded under the name of equality. Equal parental rights means that the more competitive, angrier and wealthier parent stands a better chance of winning and it is now commonplace to meet women who, desperate to leave a brutal husband, and not strong or wealthy enough to

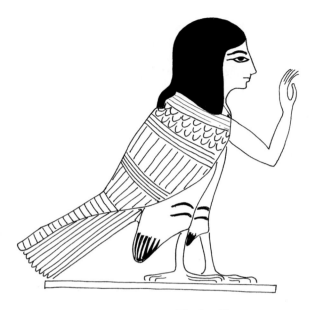

The ba. Egypt.

fight a legal battle, have opted to leave the children in the marital home and to set up alone in a bedsit or flat, a situation not far removed from the experience of women like Georges Sand and Annie Besant over a century ago who, if they were to save their own skins, had no choice but to leave their children in the custody of violent men. Just getting away from a violent marriage is achievement enough without having to defend oneself from the blows that inevitably follow.

The sanctum which was once women's natural right to retire to with their children no longer exists and in its stead we have battered wives' homes for those women brave enough to escape violence. Over centuries women who have given birth to children out of wedlock have suffered appallingly. At last after innumerable brave struggles, we have reached the point where to be an unmarried mother is no longer viewed as a sin.

Bringing up a child alone is not easy but many women now choose to do so and countless others choose not to marry their partners. However, with the stroke of a pen this could all be changed and there are strong signs that the pen might strike. It is currently being suggested that any father who registers a birth should be entitled to the same status in regard to the child as if he were legally married to the mother. In effect, this would mean that no woman, except perhaps those who choose artificial insemination, would have the right to bring up her child in her own way.

Whereas the rights of man require the dismantling of oppressive regimes in which the aristocratic few have power over the masses, the rights of woman reach deeper into the fabric of society. When women are subject to their husbands and only through them, to the state, then the oppressive regime that needs to be challenged for them is first and foremost the patriarchal family.

Democracy, as we know it, was born in Greece and is founded on the tradition of separate realms for women and men and it was not in question for women to vote. The thalamus or women's quarters was still in existence in ancient Greek times, where communities were ruled by the 'House', When democratic rights are extended to women and women, therefore, are no longer property, the God-given power of the father comes under threat. The rights of women lead inexorably to the rights of children and from there to the rights of animals, trees, plants, rivers, of the North Sea. The question then arises: does anyone have the 'right' to own anything or anyone else?

The patriarchal family is changing irrevocably and women are not likely to give up their hard-won freedoms willingly but the huge changes that society has been undergoing cause instability and uncertainty. To our ancestors our confusion would not only seem a sorry mess but a dangerous and sacrilegious trespass.

Religions and myths tell us time and again that Earth and Sky, Earth and Underworld, female and male, are separate and must remain so. When male and female enter each other's territory, so the stories say, the elements mix and the celestial bodies fall out of their orbits. The Sun falls into the Sea, the land floods, Earth and even the waters catch fire.

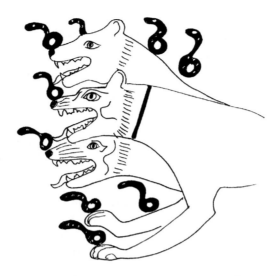

Cerebus, the three-headed hound of the Underworld.

A meditation for couples

Sit side by side, hold your partner's hand, close your eyes and
envisage a pearl between you at head level. If the pearl changes or
moves, let it.

Let your thoughts go where they will but every so often, each return
to the pearl between your heads.

After fifteen minutes or so, or when you both feel you have finished,
share with your partner what you experienced.

Eleven
Neptune   The Aura

> *'Full fathom five thy father lies*
> *Of his bones are coral made.*
> *Those are pearls that were his eyes*
> *Nothing of him that remains*
> *But does not suffer a sea change*
> *Into something rich and strange.'*
>
> William Shakespeare

It has been suggested that the tiny, dense Pluto is actually a Moon of the much larger planet, Neptune. Whether or not this is the case, it is known that the two bodies are interconnected, their oblique rotations caused by their mutual dependency. The two planets, named after the god of the Underworld and the god of the Sea, sons of Saturn, are associated with dissolution and decay. While Uranus creates the possibility of breakthrough beyond the bounds of Saturn and the limitations of the physical, Pluto and Neptune release us from the shackles of consciousness and take us through a process of transformation into a deeper and richer state of being.

When Saturn ate his offspring because it was predicted that one of them would kill him, Jupiter managed to escape and, with the encouragement of his mother, Rhea, gave his father a potion which caused him to vomit up the undigested brood. Even as a child, Jupiter was set apart; it was he who saved the entire generation and therefore the future of the Earth. This early family was not without its ups and downs and the siblings seem to have spent most of their time squabbling, the three brothers coming to blows over who should rule the world.

It was eventually settled that, while Jupiter should rule the weather and, therefore, le temps, the times, Neptune would rule the sea and Pluto, the Underworld. Their powers are constantly shifting between them: in time, earth becomes sea and sea, earth, the surface of the sea rises to become the clouds of Jupiter, which drift over the earth and shed water on the crops of their sister, Ceres, which decompose into the manure of Pluto's province. The three brothers supervise the life-cycle: conception and birth belong to Neptune in whose waters the pearl is formed and from whose seas Venus is born, while life and fate are the province of the all-powerful Jupiter, and death, atonement, repentance and redemption belong to the realm of Pluto.

They are a fraternal Mafia who do not shrink from murder, incest, rape, violence and adultery. Their sister Juno became the wife of Jupiter and the long-suffering Demeter, known as Ceres to the Greeks, while grieving the

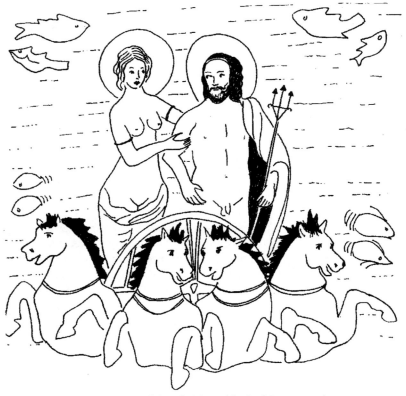

Neptune and Amphritite with the hippocampi.

144

loss of her daughter to one brother, Pluto, was raped by another, Neptune, her disguise as a mare being no protection from his consequent adoption of the guise of stallion.

Women didn't take easily to Neptune. He was a difficult, stormy character subject to sudden squalls and eddies and it was not until he married Amphridite that he began to calm down. Even then, in family tradition, he continued to seduce countless nymphs and to produce innumerable off-spring. He represents a prime energetic force whose wish is only to assert himself and extend his realm and he battles over every promontory, island and headland in his desire to engulf the earth. Ethics and morals are a later addition to the history of the world.

The spaceship Voyager confirmed the view of Neptune as a tumultuous entity, showing a planet shaken with storms. And yet, though water, sensitive to every tiny motion, can seem to rage uncontrollably, it can also be the calmest thing in the world. The salt water in our heads collects in four ventricles (the fifth contains lymph) and perhaps these are what the Sufis call the 'Four Seas'. The two lateral ventricles give access to the major and minor hippocampi that lie beneath them. The hippocampus is the mythical creature that pulled the golden shell-shaped chariot of Neptune, its body a horse and its tail a fish.

Each of the three brothers carries a trident and drives the chariot appropriate to his realm: Jupiters is pulled by eagles and Pluto's by black horses. Neptune's enabled him, as God of the Sea, to survey his realm which included inland rivers and streams as well as the oceans; as the waters of the ventricles also circulate the brain in rivulets or villi. Authors of textbooks, at a loss to know how to explain anatomical terms like 'pulvinar', 'fontanelle', 'Tree of Life', the 'three maters' or the 'thalamus' tell us simply that the pineal is so-called because it is shaped like a pine cone or that the hippocampus got its name from the creature its shape resembles. At the same time, they confess to a singular lack of knowledge of the function of these extraordinary and quite specific features of the brain. Perhaps their function is inseparable from the history and mythology of their nomenclature and, in learning to understand what it is they do, we must open ourselves to the imagination and delve into our intuition and creative mythological sensitivity as well as our academic studies.

The waters that constantly circulate our brains and spinal columns enable us to think and to perform. When the four elements are each identified with a function, water is linked to emotion, while air gets intellect; earth is allotted sensation, and fire, intuition. Emotion (water) is, then, the medium that carries thought (air) and gives it the means to be put into practice. The best way to survive a turbulent wave is to dive beneath it. The deeper you go, the calmer the water. Disturbed thoughts are inseparable from disturbed emotions and the only way to subdue them is through finding peace and silence. We cannot control water; we have to adapt to it and let go of our tension and separateness.

Water is found in many forms within the body: in, for example, saliva, blood, mucous, plasma and lymph. The lymph is a highly sensitive system running up the left side and streaming into the whole body, collecting into knots or nodes in certain areas, for instance, at the groin and under the arm. It can be envisaged as the pure, silvery, quick-flowing, spring water of the nymph, cleansing, replenishing and refreshing. When emotions are not freely expressed and released, when tension, anger or resentment are built up, the water content of the body is affected and such emotional strain can, in time, take its toll on the physical body. Orthodox medicine in the form of surgery or drugs may well rid the body of its ill effects but, even when the effects are gone, the cause may remain, the energy may still suffer, with the result that further symptoms will occur. This, of course, is frequently the case with cancer. Cancer cells in the body work with an inverted polarity system. If they are to be cured, not simply eradicated, their polarity has to be altered. Healing can only work if the healer can move beyond polarity,

attuning to the power of Neptune, the ruler of the sign of Pisces which is the last of the astrological signs and is associated with the dissolution of the individual, and whose emblem is an inverted vesica piscis, the two separating parts joined by a horizontal line.

These are the two fish of Pisces, swimming away from each other. The container, the fish vessel, is broken in Pisces, life has departed and the individual has returned to the Void.

The vesica is a symbol not only of the entrance into life but of the exit from life.

146

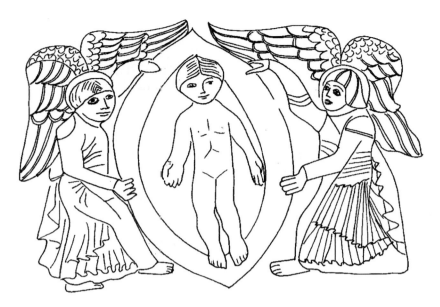

Angels guard the vesica as the soul passes through into death.

The vesica is the canal or channel that acts as a barrier and link between the worlds. It is the veil that screens consciousness from what lies beyond our ability to know. Veils used to hang in the Holy of Holies and in the Temple of Jerusalem screening worshippers from the inner sanctum. When Jesus on the cross 'yielded up the ghost....the veil of the temple was rent in twain from the top to the bottom, and the earth did quake, and the rocks rent, and the graves were opened, and many bodies of the saints which slept arose....' (Matthew 27:49-52).

To try to control emotional tensions through suppression is like trying to stay the tides of the sea. Myths associated with the Sun warn us of the dangers of ego-inflation and insist that we learn to respect the solar power at the heart of creation and myths associated with Neptune give similar warnings. Those who, like King Canute or Britannia, try to hold back or rule the waves get their come-uppance, their power cannot last. Britannia, whose influence and power derives from her status as a 'civilised' island of great navigational ability, has so prostituted her privileged position that her

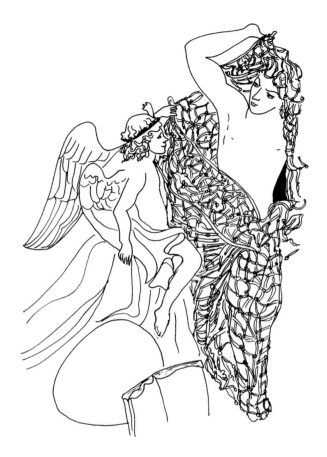

*Love (Eros) releases the soul from the net of Earthly life. Statue on an
Italian tombstone.*

seas are now the 'nuclear laundry' of the world, a misnomer that masks the
fact that there can be no clean-up.

Learning to handle the power of the Sun is the movement from the ego to
the self. Learning to handle the force of the Sea is to transcend the desire
for power and to reach an attunement with the laws of Spirit. Then, instead
of ruling or holding back the waves, one can walk over them or part the seas
at will.

Traditional descriptions of the emergence of creation from the void at the beginning of the world suggest that everything that could and would come into existence was already latently there in the waters of the deep. Sound and light, the voice and eye of God, brought it to life. Heat on cold water produces steam while air or wind lifts the condensing water into an infinite number of floating bubbles or spheres. Steam is the meeting place of heat and cold and dry and wet. It is Maya, the web of illusion, the web that is brought into being by the maioid or nymphon, the sea-spider.

In myth, the spider is Penelope, the wife of Odysseus, and her name means 'web over face'. The web over the face is, of course, the veil and Penelope was the epitome of female virtue, patience and loyalty. While her husband travelled the outer seas, she remained in the inner seas of the thalamus. To keep her suitors at bay she swore that she would not accept any of them until she had finished her weaving. Secretly, every night for seven years, she unpicked what she had woven during the day and so delayed the time when she would have to betray her husband and give herself and, therefore, her husband's House to another man.

Odysseus's story, the outer journey of war, temptation, love and heroic struggle, is recorded. Penelope's, the equally heroic mastery of the senses and devotion to an inner faith, can, perhaps, never be adequately told since it is the inner meditative process, whose web is never completed.

The web that is woven by the fertile woman and the maioid is the web of fate and of life. It is through the fertile woman that the waters of life are distributed into the future generations and through the arachnoid mater that the waters of the source are distributed through the brain, the organ of consciousness whose power of thought will produce the conditions of the

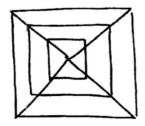

Salt forms in concentric squares around a central atom much as the pyramids were built in South America and Egypt.

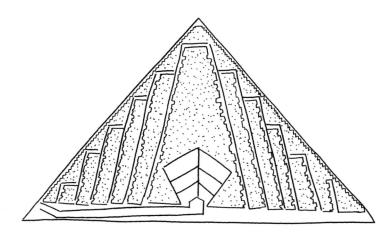

The construction of the pyramid at Suhare, Egypt.

future. Traditionally, the fertile female is hidden behind the veil, she is the other side of illusion for she is the maker of illusion. To be protected behind the web of illusion, the waters of life, is to be sheltered not only from the heat of the Sun but from the penetrating rays of consciousness and the female behind the veil is protected from the penetration of the male, and from exposure to the eye.

The thalamus is a secret place which requires respect, trust and protection. Whatever it is that lives and develops there needs time and nourishment to prepare itself for its emergence: the foetus needs the sea-waters, or albumen, of the womb to nourish it into independent life just as the cerebral cortex needs the salt waters of the thalamus to nourish its powers of thought.

Albumen is formed by salt in water so salt water not only feeds the growing chick but nourishes the human foetus. Salt water is buoyant, the word 'salt' relates to the French 'sauter', to jump. If water can be seen as the first element, the original void, which, when turned to ice, becomes quartz, the most common of all crystals whose name means simply 'ice', then salt could be said to be the first crystal formation. Salt helps to maintain the correct temperature: it melts snow, it is released in sweat to cool the body, it preserves meat and fish. In the salt sea we develop not only our bodies but our rhythm, our pulse, our heart beat. The sea gives us the means to grow into the individuals that we are but it also unites us. It is the source from which we come and to which we are always subject. To return to the source is to enter the place from which all forms emerge but which itself is without form.

White, the colour of salt, the essence, is the symbol of purity, innocence and beginnings, the colour of the virgin and the nymph who, identified with clear springs and brooks, gives her name to the white water lily or nympha. In the nymphon, or bridal chamber, the nymph is deflowered losing one flower in order to flourish into another: through experience and wisdom the simple white lily becomes the full-blown lotus or rose.

The lotus is the symbol of the attainment of paradise on Earth. Its roots form in mud, symbolically the root chakra and the element of earth, and it grows through water, the hara, then receiving the light and fire of the Sun at the solar plexus, opens into the element of air, which begins at the heart chakra, the place of transformation. The combination of all four elements takes one into the ether at the crown whose chakra opens in layers of petals above the head. As one develops in meditation, a channel of energy opens along the top of the head, Mohican-style from the bridge of the nose to the medulla at the base of the skull. The opening of this channel leads to the state of nirvana or paradise and is achieved not only by the individual who has married the two polarities within her or himself but can be arrived at with a sexual partner. The transcendence of self in both meditation and sexuality leads to a state which is sometimes referred to as 'non-being'. This is the state that Neptune takes us to, through the dissolution of the personality in the medium of water. There may be other planets as yet undiscovered but at present Neptune seems to mark the edges of the Solar System, opening the way to the stars beyond.

The state of non-being can only be reached through the blending of opposites. The fruitful union of the original opposites of 0 and I, the void and God, produce all the other manifestations of life, symbolically represented by the number 10. Two ones, eleven, form an entrance or exit, as if through pillars, beyond the manifestation of life. Extended vertically, they become the path, the way, the channel, the stream, the never-ending road to nowhere. The number eleven is the Roman number two and the Moon and Neptune have much in common; though one is our nearest heavenly body and the other is the most distant in our solar system, both

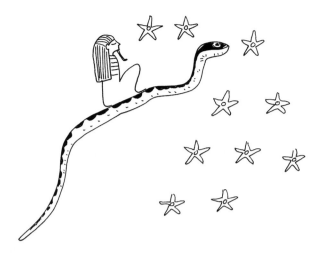

govern the seas and waters and take us beyond our conscious selves into the realm of the imagination. They give us the means to extend beyond the golden ego into the silvery unknown but, without a willing surrender of all that constitutes our identity, we flounder on the rocks of fear and, in trying to hold onto what we already know, we lose everything. Neptune dissolves us into a mystical union with the source but he also brings us up against our limitations. The parallel lines of the number eleven show a channel to the infinite but they are also the first two bars of a prison or cage.

Within tribal societies the dissolution of the individual ego and sense of separateness from other people and from the universe is aided by the ritual practices of dancing, music, chanting and the imbibing of magical potions and plants. Drug taking is a way to find union with one's soul and can be, therefore, also a healing process, helping one to be united within oneself. In our secular society, which does not recognise the human need for genuine union with others or with dimensions of life beyond our rational consciousness, we are left without any rituals to help us towards feelings of unity with other people or with God. And yet our society is overwhelmed by drugs: drugs to help us sleep, to make us forget our pain, to take away discomfort, to perk us up, to help us concentrate, to give us the means to socialise and share with neighbours and friends, drugs that break the bounds of our perceptions and drugs that take us into feelings of ecstasy and at-oneness with other people and the whole of creation.

We take drugs chaotically, with no sense of reverence, no understanding of their deeper purpose, no attempt to channel, control or develop the altered states they enable us to reach. Some drugs we term illegal while others we give out on prescription; in either case vast profits are made, indicating the value we place on drug-taking. Like any tribal society, we use drugs both to heal and to extend consciousness but we are restricted by our insistence that there is no more to life than the material: we think of health as being the absence of physical pain and we take mind-altering drugs with little more purpose than to have a good time.

To open Neptune's channel too soon or with unnatural force is to close oneself into consequent restriction. The drug addict who seeks to transcend the difficulties and pain of the physical world to a state of ecstasy must also suffer the consequent depression or downer and his bewildered loved ones suffer from the unexpected bouts of aggression and hostility that follow his unearned feelings of joy and excitement. Though he does not recognise it, he is a materialist, seeking temporary pleasure rather than eternal bliss. He is a version of Narcissus, the narcotic, addicted to himself.

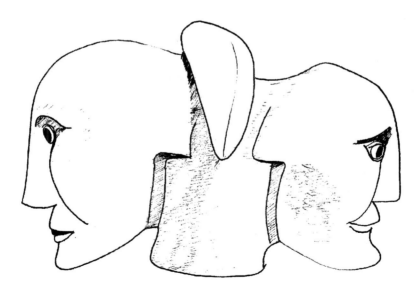

Janiform head.

The two ones of number eleven can be seen as profiles facing each other, If turned outwards, they form the two faces of Janus, the god who gives his name to January, the beginning of the year, looking simultaneously back to the past and forward to the future.

11 is the debate, the system on which we arrange our form of government, one party opposing the other in never-ending division, parallel lines destined never to meet. On its side, the 11 becomes the sign meaning equals but equality is not harmony or blend; it is an attempt to make everything the same, rather than to acknowledge and celebrate differences. The two ones can only meet if they vibrate and, through vibration, create a harmony. When a string is plucked a wave is formed which, when captured on photograph is shown as the vesica piscis:

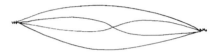

The thicker the string, the slower the vibration, the deeper the sound and the redder the colour. Energy, which is made up of electricity, sound, light and colour, passes through waves. The fish vessel joined to others of its sort makes a chain which can continue indefinitely as long as the circles from which they are formed continue to ripple, as long as the celestial lyres continue to play their harmonies.

The sign for the number one shows a pupil in an iris. Sight with the two physical eyes is dependent on polarity. The object of vision is turned upside-down on the back of the retina; it goes from positive to negative and back to positive. The interpretation of the world involves going into its

154

opposite, the mirror image contained in the void, and the optic nerves, like the aural ones, are situated behind the thalamus and the hippocampi. The two eyes working together form a single image from a blend of left and right, upside down and right-way-up, and of negative and positive.

This is the principle on which the camera works. It creates photographs and film, a flickering of images on a screen that draws us in to a world of illusion that substitutes for reality. Neptune rules not only poetry, music, dance and the mystical arts, but all that is related to film and photography. The image created by the eye and the camera is dependent on polarity, division and opposition. In seeing with the two physical eyes, we are subject to emotion. Both fear and love make us blind. We see what we want to see: the blind spot is a necessary factor in physical sight and we customarily turn a blind eye to what challenges our preconceived ideas, our comfort and security.

When the solar and lunar principles within us are balanced, when the two irises, left and right, pituitary and pineal, form a harmony, the third eye comes into being. This 'single' eye as Jesus called it, takes us beyond polarity and subjective human sight. With the third eye one sees with a clarity beyond confusion. One sees 'clairvoyantly', through matter to spirit, essence or energy. Object and subject are merged, outer and inner are combined, the intuitive and the logical are blended and what is 'seen' is also 'known'.

Christ, the Fish, was at one with the waters; and the fish-shape is the vesica, la mer/la mere, mother of the Fish. The image of Christ within the image of his mother is that of consciousness within the waters of the unconscious, solar fire within the waters of the deep. The third eye takes us to a recognition that what is permanent and real lies beyond this temporal physical world.

The transition from a belief in the solid reality of matter to a recognition of the causal and temporal nature of all things can be very unsettling and, when it hits, as it did me, with a sudden jolt, one can feel decidedly shaken up. When I was suddenly bombarded with coincidences, psychic revelations, clairvoyant flashes and other madnesses that I would happily have dismissed as codswallop if only they had let me, I felt, though I knew nothing of Neptune, 'all at sea'.

It was an unsettling time full of excitement and new openings but I felt, too, a desperate need to cling to old structures. With a head full of images of careering planets, flashing colours and dancing numbers, I found myself one day at Waterloo station looking for reading material for a journey. I must have something real and solid, I said to myself, I am too spaced out. I need to get back to some good old-fashioned, Newtonian way of thinking. So I headed for a shelf of factual blue Penguins and selected the one that looked the most serious.

On the train, I took it out of its bag. Now to get my feet back on the ground, I thought. Only then did I take in its title - *Continental Drift*. The problem is that facts, however solid and unshakeable they might appear, take you back to the only constant: everything is in a perpetual state of change. Newton, for all that we see him as father of the mechanistic world picture, was an astrologer who also practised alchemy every day for over twenty years. When, like every astrologer before and since, he was attacked for being one, he retorted, "Sir, I have studied the subject; you have not. Let that be an end to it."

The greatest scientists have always transcended the rules of science. To do so involves honouring intuition at least as much as logic, exploring the verges of consciousness, making an easy shift between the hemispheres of the brain. When the logical mind finds a harmonious balance with the spatial or intuitive, astronomy becomes astrology which encompasses both the objective view of the universe and the mythological; and anatomy takes on a depth of meaning through the recognition of the sacred nature of the human body; and so on.

In other words, solar or daylight consciousness is balanced with lunar or dream awareness. When logic sees itself as its own boss without reference to intuition or to the sacred, science is little more than hooliganism and it is hard to detect the difference between avowedly fascist science in which

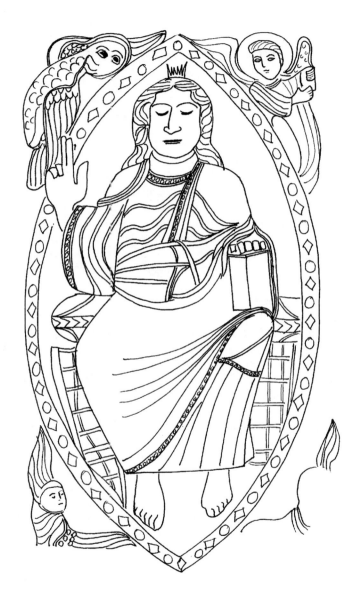

Christis in the vesica.

experimentation is inseparable from torture and what we take as normal everyday science in which, for instance, pigs are developed through genetic engineering that are so obese they cannot even stand.

Through our over-concentration on the logical, the conscious and the light of reason, we have endangered the fabric of life. We assume the right of Apollo to go the Moon just as we assume that we need more and more electric lights at night. But light pollution blots out our view of the stars, we can no longer step outside and drink in the massiveness of the universe. Because of our dependency on light we construct ever more nuclear power stations. We are afraid of the dark and cold so we create more light and heat. To do so requires the use, or misuse, of nuclear power whose waste we dump in the Earth and the Sea, the two great mothers, the forces of cold, dark and wet. The mother, whose job it is to cleanse and cradle us, to take us beyond our individual, logical minds into the realm of fantasies and dreams, to abandon the ego in favour of the universal, is abused and attacked and her power of healing undermined.

If we could learn to recognise the Earth elements - earth, water, fire and air - within ourselves and our planet, we could see when they were out of balance and recognise the warnings. The holes that are rapidly eating away the ozone layer are a direct result of the way we live, the over-concentration on the conscious mind, on the ego, and on greed. We behave, as a society, as separate beings in competition with each other. We ignore the links between us, dismiss the universe as irrelevant to us (except in that we might be able to conquer this bit or that or set up a space station on this planet or that), and treat the feminine and intuitive with disdain. It is fitting, then, that we are now suffering from the effects of too much Sun. We have chased after fool's gold, material wealth, at the expense of spiritual treasure. The ozone, the delicate layer of fine, ethereal water, cannot sustain the impact of the waste that our greed has produced. It can no longer maintain its strength as the essential filter to the Sun's rays. We are suffering the punishment of all those who, in their ambition and pride, have flown too close to the Sun. In damaging water, our mother, we are creating for ourselves a hell on Earth.

There is no such thing as matter without energy: one cannot observe a leaf without seeing its colour or smell a rose without drawing in its scent. But it is possible to sense energy without matter: we do it all the time in dreams. In sleeping and dreaming we let go of the conscious mind and of the power of the Sun, we move into the province of the Moon, the unconscious and the element of water. Water carries us beyond the individual ego and gives us the means to attune not only to each other but to other realms of existence. Just as water in the form of the atmosphere surrounds and protects the Earth, so water in the form of the aura and the etheric surrounds our physical bodies, acting as a filter and conductor for energy. The aura is a bubble, a curved film of water showing iridescent colours and responding with great sensitivity to its environment.

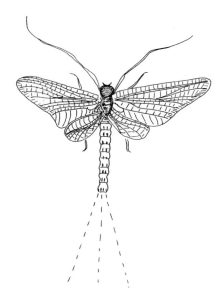

Our 'fallen' physical and emotional beings, divided into the polarities of male and female, are imperfect and subject to disease, decay and mortality. They are impermanence incarnate. The transluscent bubbles that contain us are, however, the home of the spirit, free from the decay of gross matter. 'Aura' not only means 'breath' and 'breeze'; but 'spirit' and 'Psyche', the nymph who gives her name to the butterfly or fully-fledged insect, the 'perfect form'.

Whatever is manifest in physical form on Earth is, it would seem from religious and philosophical thinking, imperfect. Perfection exists only in the imagination, where vibrations move so fast they are beyond captivity by the logical mind. The flying insect, the 'perfect form' or 'imago', hovers round our heads, fertilising the open flower at the crown. It cannot reach the thalamus, the seed bowl, but it cross-pollinates the thoughts of our brains as it flits among us through time and space. In imagery, in the imagination, we are in the realm of perfection. The 'real' world is but a poor shadow of that ideal - as anyone knows who tries to set down on paper the pure images in their head.

The imago, the imagination, can only do its job when the flower of the brain is open, when the seeds are offered on their stamens. The thalamus is a sanctum, a sacred place: receptacle of seeds, inner chamber of the brain, temple of the bee, and women's room. When both the head and the womb are honoured and celebrated for their fertility, their flowers can bloom and the imagination, the meeting place between the divine and humanity, can flourish. But when the thalamus, the women's room, is, as it is today, owned by men, it is little more than a prison, its female inmates restricted not only in their behaviour but in their thinking, their worship, their art and their ritual practice by their submission to ownership. And when, similarly, the depths beyond consciousness are subject to the rational mind, the imagination has its metaphorical feet bound and its wings clipped, and thinking is limited and distorted to fit the rules of logic.

In paying attention to the auras of our own bodies, of all living plants and creatures, of the Earth and of the planets themselves, we do homage to the spirit in matter and find meaning in what otherwise appears to be a dead universe. In acknowledging the reality of energy we give recognition to perfection, the paradisial state to which all fallen beings long to return.

Neptune shows us the ideal realm which we seem to have lost and which we can only regain through accepting the trials of life. There are no quick and easy solutions - drugs when used as escapism are no more an answer than is compulsive shopping. Reaching nirvana requires discipline: the five senses must be tuned to higher vibrations. This can only be done through accepting the imperfections of mortal life and developing compassion - for the deformed and malformed, for the old, the sick, the mad, and for one's own darkness.

The Nazis sought to reach perfection, their ideal world of fit, Aryan conquerors, through eradicating all that they perceived as physically imperfect, a horrendous perversion of the true spiritual path which does not dismiss or devalue the physical and its variety of imperfections but embraces all forms of existence with understanding and love in the knowledge that perfection can never be reached on Earth for the Earth is the testing ground where, through meeting our challenges, we gain the state of grace.

'Pluto', the name of the God of the Underworld, ruler of our darkness and corruption, also means 'treasure'. Treasure is found not only under the Earth but under the Sea and, since the Sea has once been Earth, its treasures are composed of both earth jewels and sea bounty. Amber, for instance, is the resin from ancient forests buried beneath the ocean while the pearl is formed within the sea itself.

The sea-change is the process of evolution. The study of the development of the Earth entails the examination of bones, trees, fossils and rocks (the sediment of Saturn) and, within the sea, coral is our history and geography book holding within it masses of information about the Earth and its past. But coral is suffering a similar devastating attack to that of our forests, an attack which threatens our understanding of our heritage as well as of our future, the growth, development and very survival of the life of the planet.

The entire history of the Earth lies beneath us. The past is the present intensified and compressed, fuelling and enriching us. We depend on it for our survival. No wonder that all societies throughout the world have considered it imperative to worship their ancestors and respect the Earth.

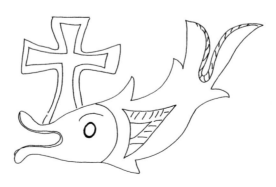

An exercise

This exercise can be done beneficially standing up. But it can also be done sitting down with feet flat on the floor.

With eyes closed, bring your awareness to the crown chakra just above the head.

From there, go up to the Individuality Point.

Come down in the aura either side of the body to a point beneath the ground and between the feet. (Like the Individuality Point, it is often surprisingly easy to contact.)

Come up through the spine and the centre of the head back through the crown chakra to the Individuality Point.

Keep repeating the process and finish after twenty minutes or so at the crown chakra.

Twelve
The Moon's Nodes
Enlightenment

'Then I saw that wisdom excelleth folly, as far as light excelleth darkness'.

Ecclesiastes 2:13

The centre of our heads is our home, the mother from which we emerge and into which we return. It is the source and the solution, beginning and end. It is the thalamus, the pool or void, the deep unconscious, the womb that contains all potential. Her child is the brain lying bean-shaped and foetus-like around her. (The broad bean, in parts of Greece, is considered sacred and may not be eaten.) The back or hindquarters of the brain is home to the ancient past, the Tree of Life, the collective history of humanity and its forebears, and is the location of the ability and need to unify, blend and balance. The front is the place of individuation and conscious thought and memory. In the back of the brain lies our collective experience, our fate or destiny, while in the front lies the possibility of individual choice and decision, the need for conscious separate development.

The front of the brain, though it may lead us on, is dependent on the back. It is at the back that the spinal fluid passes between the brain and the spine, enabling the interaction between thought and physical life. Our individual choices and ways of understanding are nothing without recognition of the past and each little step forward has been made possible only by an acceptance of what has already been. The brain is not only like a foetus but also like a continent emerging from the sea. A continent, as the word suggests, is contained and the brain is held in place by the three mothers or maters, the membranes.

As foetus or continent emerging from the womb or sea, the brain is a small mound of consciousness existing for a time above water but its days are numbered. The sea of unconsciousness laps at its shores, threatening to engulf it. Where the navel of the foetus would be is the brain's connection to the thalamus. The navel is naval or 'of the sea' and the brain is a little navigator on the waters of life.

To find guidance and direction, navigators map their voyages by the stars. Every star tells a story and each has its connections to the whole through its family or constellation. Countless myths have been associated through the ages with the stars. To plot one's life in relation to them is to recognise the archetypal significance of the mundane experiences of earth, 'to see infinity in a grain of sand'.

Life, when it is seen as a voyage with meaning and purpose, becomes a quest. A quest is both a journey towards an end and an unfolding towards a naked truth. The object of the quest is to overcome the hurdles and obstacles, to meet the tasks and to attain the treasure. Questers are always with us and are nearly always male. The female is the treasure. She is the home that is left behind and the heart or jewel that is finally attained and she is the spinner of the fates; it is she who decides whether the quester will succeed, her ability to weave being every bit as important as the questers ability to navigate or steer. While the hero sails the outer seas of consciousness and active participation, the weaver remains in deep concentration in the inner waters, conceiving, gestating and giving birth to life and to fate.

The weaver, the spider, with her eight legs and 8-shaped body, is the symbol for infinity and time. She is the Great Mother capable of both protection and deception: she protected the Prophet Muhammed from his pursuers, quickly weaving a web over the entrance to the cave in which he was hiding and so making it seem that no-one could have entered. The Prophet Muhammed, symbolically, had entered the void, the great darkness, the reality behind the veil of illusion. The spider is able to defy the laws of gravity, just as happy to walk upside-down as on the ground. From the centre of her web she moves out to all directions with equal facility, establishing the spokes on which she weaves. The centre of her web is the symbolic centre of the Earth and her eight legs when added to the four spokes of the cross of Earth, make the divisions of Earth into twelve.

The cross within the circle shows the fundamental division of space and time. It forms the basis of the compass and the clock and is a crude but necessary map and chart. The twelve radii, formed from the spider's or times eight spokes added to the cross of humanity and of Earth, give the twelve segments - of an orange, of the Round Table, of the Last Supper, of a clock, calendar and astrological chart. Twelve is the number of both time and space, of both Earth and Heaven. It shows the link between Sun and Moon and their relationship to the Earth, or central point.

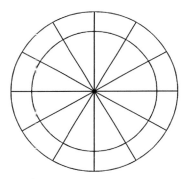

The clock is formed from the apparent movement of the Sun around the Earth; the calendar is formed from the movement of the Moon round the Earth. The balancing relationship of Sun, Moon and Earth gives us all we need to orient ourselves in time and space, to recognise the existence of the past and to see into the future. It gives us our sense of progress and development as well as our security and stability.

Like navigators, we can find our way in life by mapping and consulting the stars. To consult the rotating pattern of stars one needs a central or focal point and, in the northern hemisphere, the Pole Star, Polaris, marks the topmost point of our North/South axis. Encircling the middle of the Earth, or the East/West polarity, is the equator which, when extended into space, meets the ecliptic, the path through which the Sun appears to travel around the Earth. A child of the city and of an educational system that ignores the universe we inhabit, it was not until I was in my thirties that I discovered, through my own researches, that the Sun, Moon and planets all travel the same path. Suddenly, in recognising the perfect patterning in the cosmos, life took on an extraordinary richness of meaning. Planets are not dotted about the sky at random although, as the Earth tilts one way or the other during the seasons of the year, so the band of the ecliptic appears from our steady, central perspective, to tilt and the Sun, Moon and planets may, therefore, seem at different times to be low on the horizon or high in the sky.

Earth is not an isolated lump of rock spinning pointlessly through the nothingness of sky. It is inherently connected to the rhythms and motions of all the planets, Moons and other bodies of the harmonious whole that makes our Solar System and, beyond that, to our galaxy and, no doubt, to countless other systems of the universe.

The background to the ecliptic is a series of twelve constellations known as the zodiac. So, the Sun, Moon and planets, as they make their individual journeys at their own speeds round the Earth, can always be seen to be 'in' one of the zodiacal signs. When the wheel of the zodiac is framed around

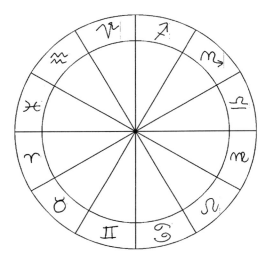

the spiders twelve divisions, or Houses, of Earth, an astrological chart is formed.

The inner part of the chart, the Houses, is spun by the maioid, the great sea spider, and represents Maya, the condition of illusion in which we live. The outer wheel, the band of the zodiac, is brought to life and illuminated by the encircling Sun, the power of light. The outer wheel shows us the form of Heaven and the inner, the form of Earth. Together, the masculine force of light and the feminine force of water provide the mists and steam that enable the wheels to go on turning.

The condition of Earth is created by the meeting of the two sexes; life is founded on polarity and it is the acceptance of polarity that gives us the means to transcend it. Polarity, the balance of opposites, gives us our orientation in space and time, it gives us the clock, the compass and the means to find guidance in the stars.

Within our heads the two vital glands, the pineal and pituitary, respond to the balancing relationship between Sun and Moon and the water content between them gives the equilibrium to the brain that we need to survive. When pineal and pituitary are in perfect balance, that is to say, when the elements of air and fire represented in the pineal are in harmony with the pituitary's elements of water and earth, the halo appears above the head. The word 'halo' is related to 'halloid', meaning a compound of salt. The halo is the symbol of spiritual attainment, it appears around or above a human being who has elevated the material level of existence to the divine. It shows the coming together of light and salt, spirit and body. 'Ye are the salt of the earth and the light of the world', Jesus told his followers on the Mount.

'Halo' is also related to the words 'hallo' and 'hallelujah'; it is a circulation of energy, an exchange of greeting between humans or between humanity and God. And halo has three specific meanings: it is the disc of the Sun, and of the Moon and it is the Threshing Floor. The three haloes, Sun, Moon and Earth or threshing floor, hang in the sky in perfect balance at the time of the harvest full Moon when the corn is cut and the wheat is sorted from the chaff. This is the Biblical Day of Judgement, the Egyptian weighing of the heart against the feather, the time when all one's actions are accounted for.

Such moments of disclosure, revelation and assessment occur when Sun, Moon and Earth make a coherent stream across the sky as if, as haloes or bangles, they have open centres which, when aligned, form a channel. The channel occurs when the regular monthly conjunction and opposition of Sun and Moon is intensified by an eclipse caused either by the Earth passing directly between the two 'lights' and casting its shadow over the Moon, or

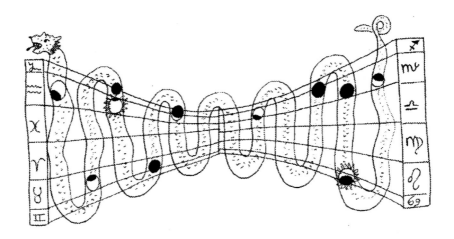

A chart for measuring the movements of Sun and Moon. The ecliptic is shown from the Tropic of Capricorn (top left) to the tropic of Cancer (bottom right) with Sun and Moon passing between them along the body of the dragon.

by the Moon passing between Sun and Earth and blotting out our view of the Sun.

For our ancestors, eclipses were of such importance that megalithic structures were built whose purpose at least partly was to honour and locate them. Full major eclipses occur only infrequently but partial eclipses occur every few months and every month Sun and Moon conjoin as the Moon appears to die and be reborn, reaching opposition a fortnight later when the full Moon directly faces the Sun. The points at which the Sun and Moon cross each others paths as they travel the ecliptic are known as the Moon's Nodes or the Dragon's Head and Tail.

The North Node is the point at which the climbing Moon crosses the path of the descending Sun and the South Node is where the descending Moon meets the path of the ascending Sun.

The South Node is also known as Cauda or the Dragon's Tail and the North Node is Caput or the Dragon's Head. Within our heads, our inner celestial domes, the two caudas weave their way between the pineal and pituitary glands just as the dragon snakes its way perpetually through the sky linking Sun and Moon. The Sun, symbolised by the dot within the circle, is the incarnating soul, consciousness itself, represented by the pupil in the iris. The Moon, shown by the vesica, is the universal mother, the sea of the unconscious, the body and the undifferentiated mass.

In an astrological birth chart, the South Node shows the position in the sky through which the soul incarnates. It shows the unconscious depths of experience or knowing that the soul brings into the individual life. The North Node shows the direction the soul needs to take to find awareness and purpose, to shed light on the depths of the soul's past. The body of the dragon traverses the sphere of the heavens or the circle of the astrological chart and shows how we can bring the experience of our lifetime to a conscious progression, how we can exit a little wiser than we entered.

These days, the standard western chart is drawn as a circle divided into twelve segments but it has not always been so. Charts have been drawn as squares, triangles, stars and other geometrical forms. The whole sky could, indeed, be represented as an arch over the Earth giving the impression of the Earth as flat. For the Egyptians, the arch of the heavens was embodied in the form of the goddess Nut who is depicted with stars extending the length of her body.

The Sun, in his different forms, passes through the body of Nut against the backdrop of the stars. When the Sun sets, he passes under the Earth and has to contend with the dark threatening waters beneath. He is accompanied and protected on this dangerous journey by his companions and is carried in a boat past the crocodiles and snakes that seek to destroy him. At dawn, having overcome all opposition, he rises again in an explosion of light.

Those who define conscious civilisation as beginning with the Greeks and Romans, dismiss the exquisite, delicate and precise art of the Egyptians and other cultures as 'primitive'. Because it is not 'scientifically' correct that the Earth is flat and the sky arches over it, earlier cultures have been considered ignorant and, even, stupid. But a 'scientific' way of seeing and interpreting is only a tiny part of a much larger whole. It is through art that we express and celebrate the divine and through symbolism that we get an intuitive understanding of cosmic forces and patterns.

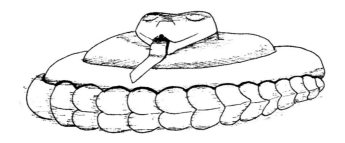

Aztec snake with thirteen coils.

The Egyptian depiction of the progress of the Sun can be understood as many voyages. It is the awakening to day and its activities, ending in the sleep of night. It is the birth of the individual, the climb to full power and maturity and the decline into death. It is the Sun's motion in one day, in one year and the duration of its cosmic life from its first explosion into life, through its greatest power to its setting or dying days as a Red Giant and its decline into a Black Dwarf.

The Black Dwarf, the night, death, the Underworld full of threatening monsters, comes at the end of the cycle of twelve. It is the number thirteen, the shedding of the old skin. The new solar year begins at the Spring Equinox when the Sun moves from the sign of Pisces into that of Aries. In the lunar calendar this is the place of the thirteenth Moon. It is Easter, the time when the Sun begins its climb towards full summer strength, the time of the birth of the Son or saviour, the resurrection after death and winter. Easter, the celebration of the cosmic egg, is a 'moveable feast', its date ascertained by the Golden Measure that marks the relationship of the Sun to the Moon.

As the Sun moves through the twelve signs of the zodiac, the solar year is completed. At the same time, the Moon's movements create the fifty-two weeks of the year. The Moon has four phases. Fifty-two divided by four results in thirteen. The solar year relates to the number 12 and is a cycle of completion. The lunar year relates to the number 13 and is a cycle of progress.

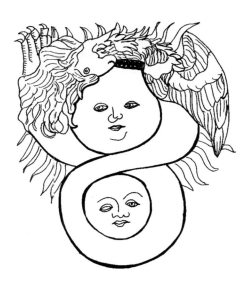

Sun and Moon joined by the dragon.

While twelve forms the circle: of the zodiac, the hours of the day, disciples, jurors and so on, thirteen draws the twelve together making the shape of the witch's, magician's or dunce's hat, and, through the central point, transforms the static wheel of twelve into a moving spiral. The central point, as a vortex, draws energies to it as well as spewing them out and provides the motion for access to another level, down or up. It can be seen in the pull of a Black Hole taking matter into anti-matter; and in the pure white spiral of the birth of a galaxy.

Where the paths of Sun and Moon cross lies the dragon, or dormant snake, the monster which in countless myths lurks in the deep, threatening to swallow the individual consciousness. Individual consciousness, the Sun, needs the protection of its fate, or Moon. The Sun without the Moon is the rampaging ego that is heedless to the guidance of higher consciousness. It will always get its come-uppance though it may, at times, be let off comparatively lightly. Jonah, for instance, who disobeyed the call of God and was tossed around on the turbulent seas of fate, was delivered back on shore to fulfil his destined task by the whale, sea-monster or dragon.

In some myths, the hero kills the dragon. But this can be dangerous. Dragons have a nasty habit of growing multiple heads or becoming yet more powerful when they are attacked. It may be better to tame your dragon, to learn to understand your ego and to listen to the guidance of the Fates. Then the snake, which was responsible for hatching the cosmic egg and releasing all the evil in the world, can come under the control of the conscious mind and can lead the individual back again to a state of grace.

The snake not only descends from Heaven to Earth but re-ascends when the time is right, elevating the plane of matter and experience to meet again with the divine. The cobra in its coiled basket is enticed upwards by the

music of the flute, instrument of Mercury or Hermes, god of civilisation, healing and regeneration. On the back of the cobra's neck is the symbol of the South Node

The cobra ascends the spine and its head arrives at a position above the human crown indicating that the human has attained the wisdom that is gained from the control of the passions.

The mortal being is at one with the divine, fulfilling its purpose on Earth, aligning itself with the motion of its cosmic snake or dragon as it winds its way between the nodes of the individual incarnation.

But what goes up must come down and the snake will descend again into the level of mud and clay, emotion and flesh, and as it does so, it will display its symbol as the North Node, the need for expression of cosmic forces in the material life of the plane of Earth.

Once again, the snake, dragon or monster of uncontrolled passion will have to be tamed as it winds its way upward through the chakras and as it wends its way across the sky touching off the relationships between the planets or gods until, passion blending with reason, wisdom is attained, full consciousness is reached, the individual soul is at one with its fate, the physical body merging with its aura or psyche. Perfection is arrived at and enlightenment strikes. This is the moment that lasts one-thousandth of a second and occurs in the centre of the head when the pineal and pituitary reach perfect balance and the halo is formed above the open crown chakra. It is depicted by the flaming pearl of wisdom revealed in the dragon's mouth, its Moonlike dew attracting the lightning of the Sun.

The pearl that is attained in enlightenment occurs for the whole Earth itself when the Sun, Moon and Earth meet in a full eclipse, when for a moment darkness covers the face of the Earth and light is reborn. The pearl that is attained in enlightenment is the wsidom that was, in fact, there all along. Wisdom, Sophia, was an active part of the process of creation from the beginning. Here she is, speaking in Proverbs 8:22-31:

> *'The Lord created me at the beginning of his work,*
> *the first of his acts of old......*
> *When he established the heavens, I was there,*
> *when he drew a circle on the face of the deep......*
> *I was daily his delight, rejoicing before him always,*
> *rejoicing in his inhabited world and*
> *delighting in the sons of men'.*

Enlightened beings return to their maker and, if they descend again to Earth, it is from their own choice, for a specific function. A re-enlightened Earth has undergone a spiritual reawakening. In the days when we human beings built massive stone monuments that aligned with the movements of the Sun and Moon and their eclipses, the renewal of light from darkness was a conscious process that aided the evolution of the Earth and all its creatures.

The fusion of Sun, Moon and Earth, the attainment of enlightenment through the eclipse of the haloes brings about the release of the soul from the plane of Earth. The busy wheel or chakra of Earth is the state of confusion, of Maya, but, through stillness, one can reach the centre, the point represented by the number thirteen, the point that is the pupil, the void of nought, the face of the deep.

Glossary

Anima Latin: the soul; the feminine that is yearned for and sought after in a male.

Animal Latin: seen by the Egyptians and others as embodying the soul; animals have been worshipped as gods in many cultures. 'To animate' is to inspirit, to endow with life.

Animus Latin: the soul; the masculine that is yearned for and sought after in a female.

Ankh Egyptian: the symbol for life.

Arachnoid mater Latin: spider mother: the middle of the three maters or meninges that surround the brain and spinal cord. Called after the spider, arachnid, because of its cobwebby appearance.

Aura Greek: breath; breeze; psyche; butterfly, golden things. The aura surrounds the living being and has different layers: the health aura is a sheath close to the body; extending beyond it is the emotional or astral level which makes up the largest part of the aura; the mental aura surrounds the head and shoulders; and the outer edge of the aura is where the qualities are found. The aura is also known as the subconscious area of mind.

Caduceus Greek: the magic healing wand of Mercury or Hermes.

Cerebellum Latin: the little or hinder brain, also known as the Tree of Life.

Cerebrum Latin: the brain, the cerebral cortex.

Chakra Sanskrit: wheel; centre. A chakra has a central point through which it draws in energy from the sun (prana or chi) and circulates it through the body and aura. There are seven major chakras situated up the centre line of the body: the root (also known as the base), hara (also called the sacral), solar plexus, heart, thyroid (or throat), pineal (or brow) and crown.

Chrysalis Greek: the gold-coloured sheath of butterflies; the state in which a larva transforms into an imago.

Coccyx Greek: cuckoo; the lowest segment of the spine resembling the bill of a cuckoo.

Dura mater Latin: hard mother; the tough, protective, outermost membrane of the three maters or meninges that surround the brain and spinal cord.

Ecliptic Greek: the circle along which the Sun passes as it appears to orbit the Earth, so-called because it is on this circle that eclipses take place.

Element Greek: simple substance of which all material bodies are composed; the bread and wine used in the Eucharist; in western tradition there are four earth elements: earth, water, fire and air. The two former tend downwards and the latter tend upwards.

Endocrine gland Greek, 'endo' means within and 'crine' means to separate: a gland which release hormones into the blood. Each endocrine gland relates to one of the major chakras: the ovaries and testes to the root, the adrenals to the hara, the pancreas (an exocrine gland, 'exe'- meaning without) to the solar plexus, the thymus to the heart, the thyroid to the thyroid, and the pituitary and pineal to the pineal or brow chakra.

Enlightenment Old English: also known as illumination. The sudden realisation of the nature of one's own life and of the nature of the universe which may be experienced as a flash of light, a bang inside the head or both.

Ether Latin: to burn or glow; the clear sky; the fifth element that unites and transcends all the others and permeates all space. In high states of meditation, the breath quickens and might even stop as we pass through the four Earth elements into that of ether.

Halo Greek: the threshing floor; the disk of Sun and Moon; a shield; the circle of light round a luminous body; the circle or disk of light around the head of divine beings.

Haloid Greek: having a composition like that of common salt.

Hara Sanskrit: soul. The hara chakra is situated below the navel and links to the adrenal glands and the release or inhibition of the hormone adrenalin. It has an orange colour and its element is water.

Heart Old English: an organ of the body; the seat of life; the soul; the spirit; the centre; the heart chakra is situated in the centre of the chest. It is the chakra of transformation, its element is air and its colour is green.

Hormone Greek: to urge on; a chemical released by one of the endocrine glands that affects the activity of a specific organ.

Hymen Greek: the god of marriage who carries a torch and veil; marriage, wedding, nuptials; the virginal membrane that stretches across and seals the entrance to the vagina in virgins.

Hymenoptera Greek: an extensive order of insects that includes ants, wasps and bees.

Imago Latin: the final and perfect stage or form of an insect after its metamorphosis. The plural is 'imagines'.

Iris Greek: goddess of the rainbow; the rainbow itself; a hexagonal prismatic crystal; a coloured membrane suspended in the aqueous humour of the eye; the inner ring of an ocellated spot on an insect's wing; a genus of plants, also called the fleur-de-lys, the heraldic lily; the narcissus.

Karma Sanskrit: the natural law that says that we must reap according to how we sow, that we receive trials and tasks or joys and rewards as our dues for past actions and as lessons for our growth. Karma extends through lifetimes.

Linga Sanskrit: the phallus, the masculine creative force.

Mandala Sanskrit: a pattern of circles and squares honouring the Sun, sometimes used for meditation.

Mandorla Greek: almond-shaped; the vesica; the ichthus; a form or pattern honouring the Moon, used in meditation.

Meditation Latin: the process of clearing the mind of extraneous thoughts to reach a sense of peace and a feeling of 'at-oneness'. There are four stages to meditation: concentration, meditation, contemplation and illumination or enlightenment.

Medulla Latin: the marrow of bones; the spinal marrow; the substance of the brain; the pith of plants; the *medulla oblongata* (elongated marrow) is the hindmost segment of the brain where the nerves cross over, linking each hemisphere to the opposite side of the body.

Nymph Greek: a semi-divine being, usually a young woman inhabiting the sea, rivers, fountains, hills, woods; a pupa.

Nympha Greek: the labia minora of the vulva.

Nymphaea Greek: the common yellow and white water lily, soul seeking birth.

Nymphon Greek: bridal chamber; a species of sea-spider.

Nymphios Greek: a male nymph.

Pia mater Latin: thin or tender mother; the delicate membrane which forms the innermost of the three maters or meninges enveloping the brain and spinal cord.

Pineal Latin: a small pine-cone shaped body situated in the head at the back of the third ventricle. It secretes melanin (*mel*: black) that darkens the skin in response to light.

Pituitary Latin: the major endocrine gland, located in the head in front of the third ventricle. It secretes pituita, also known as mucous or slime.

Planet Greek: wanderer; the planets are 'wandering stars' (as distinct from the 'fixed stars') which we see travelling the path of the zodiac as they orbit the Sun. The known planets in order from the Sun are: Mercury, Venus, Earth with its satellite, the Moon, Mars, Jupiter, Saturn, Uranus, Neptune and Pluto (although currently Pluto is nearer to us than Neptune).

Pupa Latin: an insect in quiescent state undergoing transformation into its fully-fledged form, the imago; a girl; a doll.

Reincarnation Latin: to incarnate means to clothe with flesh; to reincarnate is to return to the flesh time and again.

Root Old English, from the Latin *radix*: the descending axis of a plant or tree; the muddy base of a crystal; the part of anything that unites with something else; the root, or base chakra, is located just above the base of the spine. Its colour is red and its element is Earth.

Solar plexus Latin: *solar*: of the Sun, *plexus*: a meeting place of nerves. The chakra in the centre of the body related to the pancreas. It is yellow and of the element fire.

Thalamus Greek: the innermost part of the brain situated below the cerebral cortex and acting as a central exchange for consciousness; the receptacle of a flower containing the seeds; the temple of the bee; an inner or secret chamber; the lower deck of oarsmen on a boat; a sheep fold where lambs are nurtured; the women's rooms or sanctum. The Latin word '*gynaecium*' has the same meanings and also means a textile manufactury and the womb.

Thymus Greek: a warty excrescence; a gland that diminishes in size as we grow older shrinking to a remnant of its former self at about puberty. It is 'responsible' for building up immunity. It relates to the heart chakra.

Thyroid Greek: gateway. The thyroid chakra is located at the base of the throat and relates to the gland of the same name. It has a blue colour and its element is air.

Vesica piscis Latin: a pointed oval figure. It is formed from the overlap of two identical circles. It is often seen surrounding the figures of Christ, the Virgin Mary and the Saints. *Vesica* literally means bladder and *piscis* means fish.

Yoni Sanskrit: the vulva or external female genitals.

Zodiac Greek: a band extending either side of the ecliptic and composed of twelve constellations considered to have special influence on life on Earth and each ruled by one of the planets which, with the Sun and Moon, pass along it continuously.

Further Reading

Bailey, Alice: *Ponder on This* (Lucis Press 1971)

Baring, Anne and Cashford, Jules: *The Myth of the Goddess* (Viking 1991)

The Bible

Blurton Richard T.: *Hindu Art* (British Museum Press 1992)

Bosman, Leonard: *The Meaning and Philosophy of Numbers* (Rider 1932)

Chuang-Tzu, *The Inner Chapters, A Classic of Tao*: trans. A.C. Graham (Mandala 1986)

Dames, Michael: *The Avebury Cycle* (Thames and Hudson 1977)

Eitel, Ernest J.: *Feng-Shui, the Science of Sacred Landscape in Old China* (Synergetic Press 1984)

Frazer, Sir James George: *The Golden Bough* Macmillan 1922)

Walsch, Neale Donald: *Conversations with God* (Hodder and Stoughton 1997)

Goethe, Johann Wolfgang von: *Theory of Colours* (MIT Press 1970)

Goodison, Lucy: *Moving Heaven and Earth* (Pandora Press 1992)

Graves, Robert: *The Greek Myths* (out ofprint)

Graves, Robert: *The White Goddess* (Faber 1997)

The New Larousse Encyclopedia of Mythology.

Greene, Liz: *Saturn* (Arkana 1990)

Greene, Liz: *Relating* (Aquarian Press 1976)

Harding, M. Esther: *Woman's Mysteries* (Rider and Co.1971)

Herrigel, Eugen, *Zen in the Art of Archery* (Routledge and Kegan Paul 1953)

The I Ching or Book of Changes: trans. Richard Wilhelm (Routledge and Kegan Paul 1951)

Ibn 'Arabi: *Whoso Knoweth Himself...* trans. .T. H. Weir (Beshara Publications 1976)

Ibn 'Arabi: *Kernel of the Kernel* trans. Ismail Hakki Bersevi (Beshara)

Julian of Norvich, *Revelations of Divine Love* (Penguin 1966)

Jung, Carl Gustav: *Man and His Symbols* (Deli 1968)

Jung, Carl Gustav: *Aspects of the Feminine* (Princeton University 1982)

Jung, Carl Gustav: *Psychology and Alchemy*, (Routledge 1968)

Kemp, Martin ed.: *Leonardo on Painting* (Yale University Press 1989)

Klee, Paul: *The Thinking Eye* (out of print)

Klee, Paul: *Pedagogical Sketchbook* (Faber 1953)

Klossowski, Stanislas: *Alchemy* (Thames and Hudson 1973)

The Koran.

Lao Tsu: *Tao te Ching*, trans. Gia-Fu Feng and Jane English (Wildwood House 1973)

Lawlor, Robert: *Sacred Geometry* (Thames and Hudson 1982)

Lincoln, Bruce: *Emerging from the Chrysalis, Rituals of Women's Initiation* (Oxford University Press 1991)

Mookejee, Ajit and Khanna, Madhu: *The Tantric Way* (Thames and Hudson 1977)

Nabokov, Vladimir: *Lolita* (Weidenfeld and Nicolson 1959)

Naydler, Jeremy: *Temple of the Cosmos, The Ancient Egyptian Experience of the Sacred* (Inner Traditions, 1996)

Neumann, Erich: *Amor and Psyche, the Psychic Development of the Feminine* (Pantheon Books 1956)

O'Faolain, Julia and Martines, Lauro: *Not in God's Image* (Temple Smith, London 1973)

Rawson, Philip: *Tantra* (Thames and Hudson 1973)

Redfield, James: *The Celestine Prophecy* (Corgi 1995)

Redgrove, Peter and Shuttle, Penelope: *The Wise Wound* (Victor Gollanz 1978)

Rich, Adrienne: *Of Woman Born, Motherhood as Experience and Institution* (Virago 1977)

Rinpoche, Sogyal: *The Tibetan Book of Living and Dying* (Harper 1992)

Sacred Texts of the World, A Universal Anthology: ed. Ninian Smart and Richard D. Hecht (Macmillan 1982)

Walter (editor): *Hermetica, the writings attributed to Hermes Trismegistus* (Solos Press 1992)

Songs of Milarepa, trans Garma C.C. Chang (Shambala 1977)

Speaking of Siva trans. A. K. Ramanujan (Penguin 1973)

Steiner, Rudolph: *Colour* (Rudolph Steiner Press 1982)

Stone, Merlin: *The Paradise Papers* (Virago 1976)

The Tibetan Book of the Dead trans. Francesca Fremantle and Chogyam Trungpa (Shambala 1975)

The Vedas

Tuckett, Alice: *The Great Goddess* (dissertation 1993)

West, John Anthony, *Serpent in the Sky* (Wildwood House, London 1979)

Wilde, Oscar: *De Profundis* (Methuen and Co. 1905)

Wilson, Annie and Bek, Lilla: *What Colour are you?* (Turnstone Press 1981)

Wollstonecroft, Mary: *The Rights of Woman* (Everyman 1929)

Woolf, Virginia: *Three Guineas* (Hogarth 1986)

Yeats, W.B.: *A Vision* (Macmillan 1937)

Yeats, W.B.: *Poems* (Macmillan 1989)

Courses

Penny Allen gives individual sessions and runs courses in Meditation, Healing, Astrology and Creativity in England and France.

Tapes of meditation and healing exercises are also available.

Penny can be contacted through Capall Bann Publishing, at the address below:

> Capall Bann Publishing
> Freshfields
> Chieveley
> Berks
> RG20 8TF

FREE DETAILED CATALOGUE

A detailed illustrated catalogue is available on request, SAE or International Postal Coupon appreciated. **Titles can be ordered direct from Capall Bann, post free in the UK** (cheque or PO with order) or from good bookshops and specialist outlets. Titles currently available include:

Animals, Mind Body Spirit & Folklore
Angels and Goddesses - Celtic Christianity & Paganism by Michael Howard
Arthur - The Legend Unveiled by C Johnson & E Lung
Auguries and Omens - The Magical Lore of Birds by Yvonne Aburrow
Book of the Veil The by Peter Paddon
Caer Sidhe - Celtic Astrology and Astronomy by Michael Bayley
Call of the Horned Piper by Nigel Jackson
Cats' Company by Ann Walker
Celtic Lore & Druidic Ritual by Rhiannon Ryall
Crystal Clear - A Guide to Quartz Crystal by Jennifer Dent
Earth Dance - A Year of Pagan Rituals by Jan Brodie
Earth Harmony - Places of Power, Holiness and Healing by Nigel Pennick
Earth Magic by Margaret McArthur
Enchanted Forest - The Magical Lore of Trees by Yvonne Aburrow
Familiars - Animal Powers of Britain by Anna Franklin
Healing Homes by Jennifer Dent
Herbcraft - Shamanic & Ritual Use of Herbs by Susan Lavender & Anna Franklin
Magical Incenses and Perfumes by Jan Brodie
Magical Lore of Cats by Marion Davies
Magical Lore of Herbs by Marion Davies
Mysteries of the Runes by Michael Howard
Patchwork of Magic by Julia Day
Psychic Self Defence - Real Solutions by Jan Brodie
Sacred Animals by Gordon MacLellan
Sacred Grove - The Mysteries of the Forest by Yvonne Aburrow
Sacred Geometry   by Nigel Pennick
Sacred Lore of Horses The by Marion Davies
Seasonal Magic - Diary of a Village Witch by Paddy Slade
Secret Places of the Goddess by Philip Heselton
Talking to the Earth by Gordon Maclellan
Taming the Wolf - Full Moon Meditations by Steve Hounsome
The Goddess Year by Nigel Pennick & Helen Field
The Healing Book by Chris Thomas and Diane Baker

Capall Bann is owned and run by people actively involved in many of the areas in which we publish. Our list is expanding rapidly so do contact us for details on the latest releases.

Capall Bann Publishing, Freshfields, Chieveley, Berks, RG20 8TF